The Patient's Story

The Patient's Story

Integrated Patient-Doctor Interviewing

Robert C. Smith, M.D.
Professor of Medicine and Psychiatry, Michigan State University
College of Human Medicine, East Lansing, Michigan

Foreword by
George L. Engel, M.D.
Professor Emeritus of Medicine and Psychiatry, University of
Rochester School of Medicine and Dentistry, Rochester, New York

Little, Brown and Company
Boston   New York   London   Toronto

Library of Congress Cataloging-in-Publication Data

Smith, Robert C. (Robert Charles), 1937–
     The patient's story : integrated patient-doctor interviewing /
Robert C. Smith.
          p.   cm.
     Includes bibliographical references and index.
     ISBN 0-316-80266-2
     1. Medical history taking.   2. Physician and patient.   I. Title.
     [DNLM: 1. Medical History Taking—methods.   2. Physician-Patient
Relations.   WB 290 S658p 1996]
RC65.S65   1996
616.07'51—dc20
DNLM/DLC
for Library of Congress   95-31029
                                                                      CIP

Printed in the United States of America
SEM

Editorial: Evan R. Schnittman
Production Editor: Kellie Cardone
Copyeditor: Cathi Cote
Indexer: Dorothy Hoffman
Production Supervisor/Designer: Michael A. Granger

In memory of my first and most enduring medical influence, my father, Elmer M. Smith.

To my first teacher of humanity and so many other important things, my mother, Mary Louise Smith.

To my guide, friend, and the love of my life, my wife, Susan Sleeper-Smith.

Contents

Foreword

BEING SCIENTIFIC IN THE HUMAN DOMAIN: FROM BIOMEDICAL TO BIOPSYCHOSOCIAL

> *We include as biology not only the data obtained by observing other individuals and things, but also those that we reach through [our own inner experiences of living].*
>
> *The biologist is himself . . . of the same material of which are composed the living things that he studies.*
> **H.S. Jennings, 1933 (1)**

Biologist Herbert Spencer Jennings' early insistence that "inner experiences" are proper data for biology was my first encounter with the idea that the use of subjective data need not violate the conventional requirement for scientific respectability. Quite by chance, in 1937 as a college student, I had stumbled on Jennings' *Behavior of the Lower Organisms* (1). As a biologist, Jennings deemed his inner experiencings as a living organism no less integral for understanding living systems than his outward observations as customarily relied on for information about the physical (non-living) universe. It was, however, to be some 20 years before the complementarity of outer observation and inner experiencing fully took hold for me as a physician and helped me define the requirements for being scientific in the human domain (2–9).

As a profession and as an institution, medicine owes its origin to three distinctively human attributes. First, we humans are aware of death and its inevitability and realize that feeling and/or looking bad ("sick") may be its portent. Second, we suffer when our interpersonal bonds are sundered and feel solace when they are reestablished. Third, we are capable of examining our own inner life and experience and of communicating such to others via a spoken and written language. Critical for all three and for the work of the physician is the distinctively human capability of using words to communicate both what is being observed in the outer world as well as what is being experienced within the inner world. For each of us the distinction sick/well is preeminently manifest as inner experience, which to become known must be communicated verbally in characteristic ways. *Surely as scientists dedicated to organizing our experiences and formulating observations, we should be careful to define science in such a way as to be able to include verbal reporting as legitimate data.*

From *biomedical* to *biopsychosocial* refers to an historical transition in scientific thinking that has been taking place over the past century and a half (6). Particularly pertinent for medicine is its explicit attention to *humanness*. That alone identifies biopsychosocial as a more complete and inclusive conceptual framework to guide clinicians in their everyday work with patients. Physicians have always depended on what patients have been able to tell them about the experiences that led them to seek medical attention, testimony to the importance of verbal exchange between patient and physician being the primary source of the data required for the clinician's task. Scientists studying sick, diseased, or even dying animals or plants do not have a comparable resource; they are limited to what can be observed, as are all scientists dealing with physical or infra-human systems.

That we humans are able to participate actively in our own study by looking inward and contributing information otherwise not available should be a great scientific advantage. Yet, paradoxically, biomedical thinking, a twentieth-century derivative of seventeenth-century natural science, categorically excludes from science what patients have to tell us on the grounds of its being nonmaterial in form and not measurable; subjective not objective. On those grounds alone even posing such a question is axiomatically disallowed. Instead the human domain as a whole is seen as the art of medicine, subject neither to systematic inquiry nor possible to teach.

However, the history of medicine as far back as the papyri of Egypt 5 millennia ago documents that information provided by patients was deemed sufficiently valuable to justify writing of ways doctors might improve their skills in eliciting such (10). Paradoxically, its exclusion by medicine from medicine's science notwithstanding, few clinicians would seriously argue that what patients tell us can therefore simply be disregarded. Rather, the issue hinges on what has become a cultural imperative of western society, namely that the canons of science as defined in the seventeenth century continue to apply. The possibility that the premise itself is a fallacy is simply ignored. It is that we will now examine.

What we observe is not nature itself but nature exposed to our method of questioning.
W. Heisenberg (11)

Physicist Heisenberg's dictum exemplifies a fundamental distinction between seventeenth- and twentieth-century scientific thinking, the latter deriving from such conceptual developments as evolution, relativity, quantum mechanics, general systems theory, far-from-equilibrium thermodynamics, and, more recently, chaos and complexity theory. Loosely speaking, we are applying biomedical and biopsychosocial as labels to contrast the two positions (8).

Actually, what Heisenberg enunciates clinicians have known from time immemorial, namely, that the answers you get from a patient depend on the questions you pose and how you do so. More broadly, it exposes the fallacy of the seventeenth-century natural science position that what scientists discover exists entirely external to and independent of themselves. In fact, rather than simply examining or observing something "out there," scientists devise mental constructs of their experiences with the observed as a means of characterizing their understanding of its properties and behavior. This change in perspective began in physics with relativity theory requiring acknowledgment that the location of the observer relative to what is being observed cannot be ignored. In that transformation occurred the rediscovery of the obvious, namely, that science itself is a human activity; the lesson: that humanness and human phenomena cannot be excluded from science. Medicine's long history of successful utilization of what patients have to say about their experiencing of illness itself surely suffices to justify reviving earlier efforts at developing more systematic (i.e., scientific,) approaches to so doing.

It is important to ask questions of patients because with the help of these questions one will know more exactly some of the things that concern disease, and one will treat the disease better.
Rufus of Ephesus, 1000 A.D. (12)

To Rufus of Ephesus is credited the first formal document solely about the value of the information patients can provide. Surely his words, "will know more exactly" eloquently reveal his advocacy of an approach more scientific than those solely dependent on chance, fate, magic, or mysticism, so commonplace in those days, and still evident today in some instances of so-called alternative medicine. Rufus was revealing thereby his intuitive awareness that the very universality of sickness and death as human experiences rendered the patient a logical source of primary data.

The sick person's appeals for help and the helping responses evoked thereby already reflect a biologic social interdependency with a long evolutionary history, in humans early evident in the response to the crying of an infant. In that biologic constellation are already suggested the origins not just of sick role behavior, but also of the profession's and the institution's responses thereto. What originated in infancy as nonspecific cries of distress eventually differentiate to include personal and social awareness of being sick as a distinctive category of distress. Similarly, what may have begun merely as helping responses comes to oblige the helper to differentiate sick from other types of distress. The mother's inquiry of her child, What's wrong? or Are you feeling all right? can hardly result from anything other than learning by living and experiencing; she had already gone through the same steps herself in growing up, as have most of us.

Intuitively doctors tend to take such lay opinions seriously if for no other reason than that they often do prove to be correct. But such judgments by physicians are still mainly extensions of natural reactions we all have grown up with. They are not yet scientifically based. Biopsychosocial thinking aims to provide a conceptual framework suitable for developing a scientific approach to what patients have to tell us about their illness experiences. But to accommodate the human domain, *science* and *being scientific* must be redefined.

> *The object of science is to render as reliable as possible whatever claims to knowledge we make. . . ; [and is achieved] by reasoned efforts that ultimately depend on evidence that can be consensually validated.*
> **Charles E. Odegaard, 1986 (13)**

Historian Odegaard's succinct statement may be viewed as an effort to provide a more generic definition of science and being scientific, one independent of domain or method. With respect to the patient's verbal report of an illness experience and the doctor's version thereof, both constitute claims to knowledge about what each believes he or she knows about what happened and about what the patient's experiences were like. These constitute the data on which the doctor depends for futher study and decision-making. Doing so scientifically requires the discipline to enhance the reliability of the very process of data acquisition itself.

To explore scientific acquisition of verbal data, we can exploit the fact that every reader has surely experienced falling ill. I propose that readers pause and mentally reconstruct a recent occurrence of not feeling well, no matter how trivial, just as you might in anticipation of seeing your physician. I will do the same. But please do not look at my account until you are satisfied that what you have put together really represents what you think you would want to share with your own doctor. Our respective offerings may then be examined to see how useful Odegaard's generic definition may be for the scientific handling of what patients tell us about feeling ill. You might find it worthwhile to put your thoughts in writing, as I do now:

> *I had another of those unpleasant episodes last night. I awakened early, about 5 A.M., feeling vaguely uncomfortable. Then gradually I became aware of a steady, annoying sensation in my throat, a familiar recurring experience awakening me from sleep. The sensation is hard to describe—it is clearly located at the level of the suprasternal notch, I can indicate it with my fingers—a "full" feeling, as though somehow being stretched; slightly achy, steady; a little lump, a little sore in the throat.*
>
> *I wanted very much to sleep longer and hence tried to ignore it, but in vain. Then I realized I had slipped down from the semi-upright position and was lying flat, my head raised but slightly against a pillow. From past episodes I had learned the mitigating effects of sleeping semi-upright. I immediately sat up, swung around and, leaning forward slightly, lowered my legs to the floor. In a minute or so, I belched, with prompt relief. I lay back against the pillows, propped up at about a 70-degree angle, hoping I might now be able to sleep. But the unpleasant sensation soon returned. Determined to get more sleep, I did the next thing that usually helps; I got up and, while standing and moving about, drank a few swallows of hot water. Soon came the first of three belches and again prompt relief.*
>
> *Confident that I would enjoy another couple of hours of sleep, I returned to bed, again propped up. I awakened symptom-free, but feeling a little sad, remembering how in the past when my wife had noticed I had slid down, she would try to help me get repositioned before symptoms developed. She has been in a nursing home for more than a year.*

A representative sample of human (patient-derived) data, however idiosyncratic, how may its acquisition and processing be rendered as scientific as possible?

> *[The scientist] devises mental constructs of his experiences with [nature] as a means of characterizing his understanding of its properties and behavior. . . . [They, in turn,] are predominantly communicated by language, it being difficult to communicate them in any other way than by speaking about them.*
> **M. Delbruck, 1986 (14)**

> *The whole of science is nothing more than a refinement of everyday thinking.*
> **A. Einstein, 1950 (15)**

The raw data patients proffer are in the form of speech, gesture, and posture, and not much else, that is, bits of distinctively human behavior, verbal and non-verbal. Physicists Delbruck and Einstein remind us of two things: that twentieth-century conceptual transformations render self-evident the dependence of *science* and *being scientific* on a spoken and written language, and that the efforts of the person feeling sick to figure out what is happening call on the same mental operations humans ordinarily employ whenever confronted with threats to their sense of well being. But in contrast to the distress evoked by threatening external events or circumstances, feeling sick and falling ill more often begin as private experiences not necessarily knowable to anyone else. Hence the truly scientific physician not only must access that private world, but also must be reasonably assured that the information (data) can be relied on. Critical is recognition that the patient is both an initiator and a collaborator in the process, not merely an object of study. The physician in turn is a participant observer who in the process of attending to the patient's reporting of inner-world data taps into his or her own personal inner-viewing system for comparison and clarification. The medium is dialogue, which at various levels includes communing (sharing experiences) as well as communicating (exchanging information). Hence, *observation* (outer viewing), *introspection* (inner viewing), and *dialogue* (interviewing) are the basic methodologic triad for clinical study and for rendering patient data scientific (9).

My written account of illness provides an opportunity to examine a patient's inner viewing not yet influenced either by the physical presence of, or by dialogue with the doctor. It derives both from what I literally strove to remember and reconstruct of what I had experienced a couple of hours earlier, as well as from much else that came into my mind in the course of so doing. The actual, written material available to the reader, however, is already limited by the fact that I am obliged to convey that information not only in words but in writing, and in a textbook to boot. Moreover, you have no means to ascertain on what basis my final words were selected from the myriad of associations with which I was bombarded in the process of its writing. Clearly this process is very different from what would have gone on in my head were I seated in the doctor's waiting room rehearsing what I would want to tell him.

Such a state of affairs at once identifies long-known barriers to being scientific in the handling of human (patient-derived) clinical data. Painfully evident is it that what can be communicated of such data to others is limited both by the frailty of human memory and the constraints imposed by the requirement to convey in words experiences for which suitable words may not exist. Gaps are inevitable, between what patients experience and what they can effectively communicate to the doctor; between the words of the patient and what the doctor remembers and may select as relevant; and ultimately between the preceding and what the doctor ultimately reports orally or writes in the record, the public record of data available for clinical reasoning.

Yet the fact remains that notwithstanding such formidable obstacles, experienced clinicians using observation, introspection and dialogue can be remarkably successful in documenting the existence of explicit pathologic bodily processes and associated non-disease issues, first inferred simply from what the patient had to say. Thus a clinician knowledgeable about physiology, surely would quickly consider problems with the esophagus as one plausible explanation for the attacks I describe and would accordingly pursue appropriate inquiries to test such an hypothesis (16). Moreover, the experienced clinician would recognize the interrelationship of my disease process and my personal life. Consider, for example, how my sadness about my wife's incapacity might affect my esophageal symptoms; for example, worse since she went to the nursing home.

Biomedical education's a priori assumption that such patient-derived data and the means of their acquisition are neither teachable, nor subject to systematic study, needs to be examined. To do so let us consider two dimensions of such data, again using my case protocol.

> [The] relationship between doctor and patient partakes of a peculiar
> intimacy presuppos[ing] on the part of the physician, not only

*knowledge of his fellow man, but sympathy . . . [D]esignated
as the art [of medicine] . . . [intimacy], should most properly
be called [its] essence.*
W. T. Longcope, 1932 (17)

*[The] widened, vicarious experience [provided by] narrative is
memorable precisely because it is necessarily enmeshed with past and
future, cause and consequence.*

*[Patients'] life stories cultivate . . . interest in their oddities and their
ordinariness—and a tolerance of both. . . .*

*The narrative in each case belongs to a human being who is an object of
scientific study and to that person's world of lived experience and
belief. . . . [It] remains central to knowledge in medicine [precisely]
because the patient is the focus.*
K. M. Hunter, 1991 (18)

Odegaard proposed defining *science* as independent of domain
(13). But a universal requirement for being scientific is that we
understand and respect the natural state of whatever domain we
are concerned with. Thus, just as marine biologists must master
functioning underwater to study marine life scientifically, so too
must clinicians accommodate to what is distinctive about the
human condition and the environment of patients. And what is
more distinctive about being human than how we communicate
and interact?

In effect, Longcope's "intimacy" refers to a unique quality of the
doctor's relationship with the patient, one he felt so indispensable
that medicine "would cease to be" medicine without it. Where in
my protocol, if anywhere, does *intimacy* reveal itself? I know,
because in my anticipation of meeting with my doctor, I deliberately included one item which on the face of it would seem to
contribute little or nothing to his understanding of the symptom
complex I was struggling to make clear to him. (Actually it had
contributed something, as already mentioned.) It was my reference
to my wife's being in a nursing home. His response to that in-
tensely personal and poignant item would, I anticipated, give a
clue as to where we stood with each other, whether my confidence
in our *intimacy* was shared by him.

By the same token, while imagining myself telling my doctor
what I had just gone through, my recollections quite naturally took

on a narrative form, as my story. That is, after all, how we humans ordinarily communicate our experiences to others, especially those to whom we would turn for help. As Hunter reminds us, narrative style facilitates vicarious participation of the listener in whatever the patient was or is experiencing. That in itself implies an element of intimacy between the two participants and helps direct attention to what is distinctive about the individual whose story is unfolding.

Readers need only review their own experiences with doctors taking [*sic*] their histories to appreciate the difference between encouraging narration and requiring reporting. The latter approach is deliberately interrogative, the doctor assuming the initiative and agenda, the patient, an object of study rather than an active participant in his own study. Eighteen seconds has been reported to be the mean length of time to elapse before doctors interrupt the patient's first response (19). Small wonder patients complain that doctors don't listen. Interrogation generates defensiveness, narration encourages intimacy.

But do the words intimacy and narration refer to phenomena about which consensual agreement with regard to criteria can be achieved? The answer to that question is key to whether the concepts the words express fall within the scope of science. The history of science is a record of repeatedly rendering the tacit manifest, the difficult easy, the impossible possible. We all agree the answer to our question is difficult, for many reasons already cited. Others insist the very consideration of such questions in medical matters to be impossible. But characteristic of science also is surprise, the unexpected—a sudden discovery or technologic development in one field that fosters a corresponding progress in another.

> . . . [R]ejoice in the discovery of a great and final instrument of drama [one], which all the other arts have had since time immemorial, which the oldest art, the theatre, lacked until today; . . . [an] instrument that gives it precision and scientific serenity.
> **R. Boleslavsky, 1933 (20)**

What discovery could be so important to a noted stage director and teacher of acting to inspire him to announce it as finally providing the theatre "precision and scientific serenity"? Astonishingly, Boleslavsky awarded that high honor to the newly introduced "talkie" motion pictures, at that very moment being ridiculed by traditional theatre as an outrageous degradation of the stage and its art purely for commercial purposes. For Boleslavsky films finally made possible the preservation of the art of the actor and of the theatre. "Do you realize," he passionately exclaimed, "that with the invention of spontaneous recording of the image, movement and voice, and consequently of the personality and soul of an actor, the theatre is no more a passing affair but an eternal record?"

Written more than 60 years ago, Boleslavsky reveals an impressive grasp of one of the essentials of being scientific, namely, to have publicly available and lasting records of natural phenomena otherwise evanescent or not accessible to direct human perception. The introduction of talkies, an early stage of audiovisual (AV) technology, marked the first time in history that humans could observe the behavior not only of another but of one's self, and do so repeatedly and in public! Though I have made use of AV technology for teaching and research for almost 50 years, appreciation of that momentous change for humankind came to me only on reading Boleslavsky's *Acting. The First Six Lessons.* *

The conclusion seems inescapable. However powerful the cultural imperative engendered by the seventeenth-century scientific revolution, medicine's resistance — or more accurately, blindness — to the need to address the issue of being scientific with human data stems not just from the inherent difficulty of so doing, but from a lack of any dependable means to do so, an altogether common occurrence in the history of science. For the human domain AV technology fills that gap just as did telescopy for astronomy and microscopy for biology.

A successful dialogue between patient and physician is at the heart of working scientifically with patients.
G. L. Engel, 1995 (21)

Those words epitomized my final tribute to John Romano (1908–1994); they also epitomize this book. What they recall is the impact of my seeing Romano in 1941 sit down with a patient on medical rounds and engage with him as though in the privacy of his office. That single experience was to inaugurate an association between us that culminated in Romano's concept of human biology (22) and

---

*When I first came upon Boleslavsky's little "dialogue" with the fictional "Creature," an inexperienced, stagestruck young ingenue in 1992, it seemed to me that both he and I had been struggling with the same problem: his concern, how to teach actors; mine and my colleagues, how to teach medical students; the common domain, *human phenomena not subject to re-examination.* G. L. Engel, 1995 (21)

my move *beyond* the biomedical to the biopsychosocial, finding synthesis and subsistence in the Rochester medical curriculum as an integrating, driving reality. Bob Smith's book represents an effort to extend that reality by examining its operation at the very heart of the doctor-patient encounter in the process of the interview.

The Patient's Story: Integrated Patient-Doctor Interviewing makes progress in key areas although such a claim becomes possible only after we see how the book works in students' and other learners' hands. In final analysis research on how effectively learners pick up this approach will be important (23), as will the impact its patient-centeredness has on the patient (24). For example, can it be shown that patients feel better, or do better, when the interviewer uses this approach (24)?

Identifying a basic infrastructure of the interview carries much potential for medicine as a science. The benefit, of course, is that a basic interviewing approach allows us to obtain human data in a more systematic way—by one interviewer on multiple occasions or across many interviewers. To the extent successful, this addresses Odegaard's concern that as a means of acquisition of data the interview process be demonstrated as reliable as possible. Smith's emphasis on how idiosyncratic and confusing approaches to teaching interviewing to students have been in the past is well taken. The lack of a basic methodology to medical interviewing may itself have encouraged students to acquire patient data erratically and unsystematically. While providing sufficient structure and necessarily detailed instructions for the beginner, the overall approach is still flexible enough to offer promise that the personhood of the patient and the humanity of the interviewer will both be enhanced.

As Smith cautions, this interviewing approach must not be seen as a final destination for the interviewer, but rather as a point of departure. This prospect is facilitated by the text's incorporation of teaching directed specifically at enhancing the doctor-patient relationship, especially by fostering the effectiveness of the intimacy between doctor and patient; by considering introspection at the level of better understanding oneself and the importance of opening such self-awareness to the patient; and by actively incorporating the relational dimension of interviewing instruction and placing it on equal footing with the informational aspects of interviewing.

An important distinction this book makes, often overlooked or misunderstood, is that while the biopsychosocial model provides a basis for the description of the patient and the patient's problems, the ability to interview effectively is indispensable for operationalizing the model, hence my earlier reference to the significance of a "successful dialogue."

George L. Engel

References

1. Jennings, HS. *Behavior of the Lower Organisms*. New York: Columbia University Press, 1923. Pp. 14, 22.
2. Engel, GL. "Homeostasis, Behavioral Adjustment, and the Concept of Health and Disease." In Grinker, R, *Mid-Century Psychiatry*. Springfield IL: Charles Thomas, 1953. Pp. 33–59.
3. Engel, GL. Selection of clinical material in psychosomatic medicine: The need for a new physiology (Special article). *Psychosomatic Medicine* 16:368–373, 1954.
4. Engel, GL. A Unified Concept of Health and Disease. *Perspectives in Biology and Medicine* 3:459–485, 1960.
5. Engel, GL. *Psychological Development in Health and Disease*. Philadelphia: Saunders, 1962.
6. Engel, GL. The need for a new medical model: A challenge for biomedicine. *Science* 196:129–136, 1977.
7. Engel, GL. The clinical application of the biopsychosocial model. *Am J Psychiat* 137:535–544, 1980.
8. Engel, GL. How Much Longer must Medicine's Science be Bound by a Seventeenth Century World View? In White, K.L. (ed.), *The Task of Medicine: Dialogue at Wickenburg*. Menlo Park CA: Henry J. Kaiser Family Foundation, 1988. Pp. 113–136.
9. Engel, GL. On looking inward and being scientific. A tribute to Arthur H. Schmale, M.D. *Psychotherapy and Psychosomatics* 54:63–69, 1990.
10. Sigerist, HE. *A History of Medicine. Vol I. Primitive and Archaic Medicine*. New York: Oxford University Press, 1951.
11. Heisenberg, W. *Physics and Philosophy. The Revolution in Modern Science*. New York: Harper, 1958. P. 58.
12. Sigerist, HE. *Op. Cit.*, Pp. 326–327.
13. Odegaard, CE. *Dear Doctor. A Personal Letter to a Physician*. Menlo Park, CA: The Henry J. Kaiser Family Foundation, 1986.
14. Delbruck, M. *Mind from Matter? An Essay on Evolutionary Epistemology*. Palo Alto: Blackwell Scientific Publications, Inc., 1986. P.251.
15. Einstein, A. *Out of My Later Years*. New York: Philosophical Library, 1950. P. 59.
16. Gignoux, C, Bost, R, Hostein, J, et al. Role of upper esophageal reflex and belch reflex dysfunctions in noncardiac chest pain. *Dig Dis and Sciences* 38:1909–1914, 1993.

17. Longcope, WI. Methods and medicine. *Bulletin, Johns Hopkins Hospital* 50:4–20. 1932.
18. Hunter, KM. *Doctors' Stories. The Narrative Structure of Medical Knowledge.* Princeton, NJ: Princeton University Press, 1991. Pp. 17, 124, 129, 155.
19. Beckman, HB, and Frankel, RM. The effect of physician behavior on the collection of data. *Ann Int Med* 101:692–696, 1984.
20. Boleslavsky, R. *Acting. The First Six Lessons.* New York: Theatre Arts Books, 1962.
21. Engel, GL. "For whom the bells toll a second time. John Romano, physician and psychiatrist (1908–1994)." *Rochester Medicine.* University of Rochester, Summer 1995, 10–12, 36.
22. Romano, J. Basic orientation and education of the medical student. *J Am Med Assoc* 143:409–412, 1950.
23. Smith, RC, et al. Improving residents' confidence in using psychosocial skills. *J Gen Intern Med* 10:315–320, 1995.
24. Smith, RC, et al. A strategy for improving patient satisfaction by the intensive training of residents in psychosocial medicine: a controlled, randomized study. *Acad Med* 70:729–732, 1995.

Preface

I designed *The Patient's Story: Integrated Patient-Doctor Interviewing* for students who want to learn how to interview patients. I heard a common message when I asked students for guidance while writing this text. Students have been told how important the doctor-patient interview is but are disappointed and frustrated by its teaching. Upon completion of initial training, most students say they know a few separate skills, but they do not know how to put them together into a coherent interview. Some students also ask, in one way or another, "If the relationship is so important, why don't you teach us how to develop it instead of simply telling us that it's important?" And others, "You seem to be telling us that all there is to the relationship is being nice."

During the last 15 years I have developed a teaching method that responds to students' concerns. This method first required building on existing advances to synthesize a unified interview. I was then able to describe "how" to perform this interview on a step-by-step basis.

The clarity required to describe an interviewing process that includes both the informational and relational aspects of communication obliged me to write a detailed and specific book. Fortunately, systematic guidelines make the student's job easier. Moreover, these guidelines do not require that one interview inflexibly or by rote. Rather, this book provides an infrastructure as a starting point. The student can then better deploy her or his own rich and varied style to understand the unique aspects of an individual patient.

I planned the text for medical students: preclinical students beginning their interviewing careers and clinical-level students who are trying to put it all together. Nevertheless, the book adapts well to the needs of other learners (and their teachers) where interviewing and the doctor-patient relationship are central: housestaff, practitioners and faculty, nurses and nurse practitioners, physician assistants, behavioral scientists, dentists, and other health-care givers.

The book works best used in the order presented. Chapter 1 orients the student to interviewing, provides necessary background material, and presents an overview of Integrated Patient-Doctor Interviewing, the unified interviewing approach presented in this book. Chapter 2 describes individual interviewing skills, which are synthesized in Chapter 3 as the patient-centered process of Integrated Patient-Doctor Interviewing. Chapter 4 outlines symptom-defining skills, which are then synthesized in Chapter 5 as the doctor-centered process of Integrated Patient-Doctor Interviewing. I recommend that students focus first on the patient-centered dimension of the interview and later incorporate the doctor-centered dimension. Chapter 6 considers many practical issues for fine tuning Integrated Patient-Doctor Interviewing. Chapter 7 addresses the second determinant of an effective interview, the doctor-patient relationship, with a focus on interviewer self-awareness, patient personality types, and nonverbal communication. This material is relevant in both beginning and clinical-level interviewing. Chapter 8 describes how interviewers present the information obtained from the patient and, in turn, present it to others verbally and in writing. Chapter 9 describes how one gives different types of information to the patient, a skill best learned after students have gained facility with basic interviewing.

I wrote this book intending that the student gain an expertise with interviewing that will match her or his facility with the anatomy of the hand, the Krebs cycle, the physical examination, and the differential diagnosis of chest pain. My greatest hope is that students become aware of the remarkable beauty and simplicity of the interviewing process, that they understand how effective communication unites student and patient, and that they experience this process as the route to better understanding themselves as well as their patients.

R.C.S.

Instructor's Preface

Because *The Patient's Story: Integrated Patient-Doctor Interviewing* presents a somewhat different approach to interviewing, a companion teaching supplement is available for teachers and other interested faculty. We originally had planned to include the teaching supplement in this text but received feedback that combining material for teachers and students did not work well.

The teaching supplement considers how teachers might teach the new material presented in this book. It extensively details one way to teach beginning medical students the patient-centered interviewing approach—in 10 sessions, each with a 1-hour lecture/demonstration followed by a 2-hour skill-oriented small group experience. The teaching supplement also describes in considerable detail how one can teach personal self-awareness to students (and others) and how to integrate self-awareness training into the 10-session patient-centered interviewing course just mentioned.

The 61-page supplement is available from the author for a prepaid $15 charge: Robert C. Smith, B306 Clinical Center, East Lansing, MI 48824. I also invite questions and feedback at this address or via E-mail: 21770rcs@msu.edu.

Acknowledgments

This text really started when a friend and colleague, Ruth B. Hoppe, suggested that I put my interviewing instructions in writing. Our 1991 article, "The Patient's Story: Integrating the Patient- and Physician-Centered Approach to Interviewing," was the beginning. Subsequently, Kimberly Kist and Evan Schnittman at Little, Brown asked me to expand this approach into a book. Their encouragement, and Evan's later feedback and devotion to quality, provided key support and direction as I wrote about a different approach to teaching medical interviewing.

I was blessed to receive assistance with the manuscript from two incomparable professionals who provided helpful feedback in many areas, curbing my urge to get on with things and encouraging me to create a text that was both user-friendly and meaningful. Both have had a significant impact on my personal and intellectual development in the past, and our work on this text became a happy extension of that process. George L. Engel, who wrote the foreword to the book, provided help that stimulated and clarified my thinking in many areas, especially about how interviewing influences the scientific nature of medicine. He also helped me clarify language and definitions in many ambiguous areas. Mack Lipkin, Jr. provided a thorough, painstaking look at the manuscript, making suggestions that greatly improved the integrity and consistency of several concepts. He pointed to the need for greater precision in some areas and less rigidity in others, and to the importance of better balance in still other areas. As always in working with Mack, I learned about myself.

Fred Platt assisted with the final editing chores. Not only did I learn much from him, but I appreciated the timely, supportive way in which he made his contributions and the significant improvement in readability that occurred. Fred also added important conceptual input, particularly in the development of a separate health issues category.

These colleagues and friends deserve much credit for any success of this book. The responsibility for shortcomings in the book, however, lies squarely on my shoulders.

Feedback from faculty, students, and residents also was essential. Each chapter was read by faculty colleagues here, at Michigan State, and elsewhere. Members of our Psychosocial Teaching Group and our Psychosocial Research Group provided significant input at the early, formative stages that helped shape the book. I will be forever indebted to the students in my mentor group, my doctor-patient relationship group, and several of my interviewing groups. These first- and second-year students helped me achieve the clarity students require, often providing valuable feedback in unexpected areas. Similarly, our first-year residents in internal medicine and in family practice provided superb feedback, as did several of our senior medical residents. The students and residents not only provided useful critiques of the text but also were the proving grounds for teaching and learning interviewing in this way. There is not room to name all my faculty and learner colleagues who gave so much of themselves and their time, but the book could not have been done without their help.

My secretary, Bonnie Zell, provided valuable input and suggestions and shared her remarkable artistic skills with the graphics.

It would be a serious oversight if I did not mention several more remote but nonetheless critical influences on this book. My own growth and learning in psychosocial medicine began in the biopsychosocial programs at the University of Rochester. Tremendous personal and professional awakening occurred with my introduction to the true nature of patients — and to myself. My journey was then fostered by the American Academy on Physician and Patient. Further learning and personal growth could not have happened without many wonderful friends and skilled professionals. I also have been strongly influenced by the Fetzer Institute where I have come to better understand the role of spirituality in medicine — and patients' suffering and quest for meaning in their lives. During the last 10 years, it has been my great fortune to be at Michigan State University where the atmosphere is truly biopsychosocial. It simply is part of the university's culture. My work could not have occurred without this propitious milieu and, of course, the many here who epitomize and live the integration of mind and body in their personal and professional lives.

I want to acknowledge, in closing, many equally powerful influences and teachers: my patients.

The Patient's Story

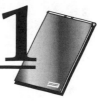

Interviewing

How are you feeling? Are you sick? We humans know when something is wrong but how do we convey our problem—and how does the medical student diagnose the problem? The student learns what is wrong by interviewing the patient and identifying his or her symptoms and personal concerns [1]. Although uniquely private and subjective, symptoms and concerns are the primary data—the hard data of the science of medicine—and we can enhance their scientific value through good interviewing.

These human data lead to most diagnoses and determine most treatment [2–6]. By *human data*, I mean information that the patient communicates in words or through nonverbal but uniquely human modes of expression, for example, a frown. These data are found in no other domain. For example, height, weight, an enlarged liver, an elevated cholesterol, or a high blood sugar, observed directly or indirectly by the interviewer, is not a uniquely human datum. But a patient's report of a symptom or personal concern is uniquely human information. Human medicine is the only scientific field in which the subject literally tells the scientist what the problem is [1]. A diseased plant or animal, a collapsing rock structure, or an aberrant molecule cannot. If the science of medicine was similar to these, the doctor would simply perform a physical examination and run some tests. I offer a challenge to the student: Keep human data foremost and do not rely primarily on the physical examination or laboratory tests. Interviewing is the key skill of the physician. The data obtained markedly enlarge the scope of medical science.

Most students enjoy interviewing. Interviewing launches their clinical careers and often provides the brightest spot in the first two years of medical school. Interviewing puts the student at the heart of medicine—working with a patient. To be certain, seeing a patient for the first time may provoke anxiety, but living the reality of becoming a physician far outweighs the fear. Most students say something to this effect: "Now I'm beginning to see where all this basic science stuff is going, I'm starting to see the light at the end of the tunnel."

Although it is difficult to master interviewing, students possess many necessary skills. Not only have they cleared multiple hurdles to get this far in their careers, but they bring a life-long experience of communication. Students also have many interpersonal and relational skills, which are among the most important skills required for successful interviewing. Nor are students completely unfamiliar with the vicissitudes of life that patients will present. Students do not come unprepared, but need to further develop their existing expertise in the medical setting and learn some new skills.

Interviewing is an exchange of relevant information about the patient for the interviewer's professional purposes. Why is interviewing so important [7,8]? First, it is the vehicle for the interaction and exchange of information in nearly all circumstances. Second, the greater part of information about a patient comes from the interview [2]. In fact, interviewing produces data needed for diagnoses more often than the physical examination and laboratory investigation combined [3–6]. Third, interviewing generates most data essential to treatment and prevention and is the major vehicle by which information of all types is transmitted to the patient [9]. Finally, and probably most important, interviewing itself determines how the doctor-patient relationship evolves [9]. Conversely, the quality of the relationship with the patient influences the quality of data exchanged [10,11]. Note that clinicians perform from 120,000 to 160,000 interviews during a career [12]. Sir William Osler captured the role of the interview long ago when he said, "By historical method [the interview] alone can many problems in medicine be approached profitably. [13]" Interviewing is worth doing well and efficiently [2].

In sum, interviewing is the most fundamental of all medical skills. Not only does it provide most diagnostic and therapeutic information about the patient but it also is the major determinant of the doctor-patient relationship and outcome of care. Nothing in medicine requires greater expertise and mastery than this skill, the core skill of medicine.

Integrated Interviewing Permits the Student to Synthesize the Biopsychosocial Story

The focus of this book is an interviewing approach that elicits relevant personal and symptom data about the patient. After obtaining these human data, the student synthesizes them into a description of the patient—their biopsychosocial story.

The Biopsychosocial Model

The biomedical model (also known as disease model, biotechnical model) describes patients only in terms of diseases, psychiatric as well as physical, and excludes most psychological and social aspects of the person [14,15]. Although responsible for many of medicine's successes, the biomedical model has also caused much damage by ignoring the human dimension, and now is evolving into a biopsychosocial model.

Doctor George L. Engel proposed a biopsychosocial model to describe a person as an integrated mix of her or his biological, psychological, and social components [16,17]. Because this model integrates the psychological and social dimensions with the biomedical aspects, it is both a humanistic and a scientific model for medicine [9]. The biopsychosocial model includes the person with the disease as well as the disease; for example, the unique personal features of the patient, the doctor-patient relationship, the family, the community, and the spiritual dimension [9,10,16–20]. This is a roundabout way of saying that the mind and body are not separable and that the modern caretaker can best understand the patient only as a whole person [10].

Yet students often become frustrated with the biopsychosocial model. Students observe that the biopsychosocial model itself "doesn't give a clue" about how to obtain the biological, psychological, and social data the model prescribes. Engel's model identifies content without addressing the interviewing process by which one elicits data necessary to synthesize that content.

The Interviewing Approach

Students trained in the biomedical model are taught to elicit symptoms of disease by using a "doctor-centered" interviewing process. *Doctor-centered interviewing* means the student or physician takes charge of the interaction to meet her own needs to acquire the symptoms, their details, and other data that will help him identify a disease. By eliciting many bits of these nonpersonal data, the student can synthesize them into a description of the patient's disease. Personal concerns are largely ignored and discouraged so that the student can isolatedly focus on making a disease diagnosis. A doctor-centered interview thus takes the lead away from the patient and prevents most personal information about the patient from arising, limiting the interviewer's ability to develop an adequate psychosocial description [14,15,21,22].

To correct this, a new process that generates personal data has evolved—"patient-centered" interviewing [23–29], also called a "relationship-centered" approach [29]. *Patient-centered interviewing* means that patients are encouraged to express what is most important to them. In addition to symptoms, they can express their personal concerns. By also eliciting these personal data, the interviewer can synthesize a psychosocial description of the patient. Not only does the interviewer avoid an isolated focus on symptoms, but she or he also allows the patient to lead and direct the conversation to important personal data, usually the personal context of the patient's symptoms and disease [10]. The patient's ideas and concerns, rather than the doctor's, are paramount. Patient-centered interviewing was developed to complement doctor-centered interviewing; I do not recommend its use in isolation.

The issue is not which process is best. We need both. Integrated Patient-Doctor Interviewing, the focus of this book, combines patient-centered and doctor-centered interviewing processes to elicit both personal and symptom data. Students must then interpret and synthesize these data, using their knowledge of medicine, along with available data from physical examination and the laboratory, to produce a biopsychosocial description—the patient's story [9].

The term *patient-centered* can be used in two ways. In a general sense, every action with the patient is patient-centered because everything is done in the patient's interest. Confusingly, one of the processes to achieve this also has been termed "patient-centered interviewing" to contrast it to "doctor-centered interviewing." Rather than introduce new terminology, these terms will suffice as long as the student recalls that both processes ultimately are employed toward meeting the patient's needs.

In sum, the biopsychosocial model describes the patient and Integrated Patient-Doctor Interviewing serves to obtain the human data that the student can then synthesize to make a biopsychosocial description.

Clinical Approach

With Integrated Patient-Doctor Interviewing, the patient's needs always take precedence [23–27]; the interviewer should recognize that a patient can have many different needs, as detailed in Table 1-1. Before the interview is begun and during its early parts, the interviewer scrutinizes the patient for obvious symptoms of an

Table 1-1. Needs communicated by patients

Needs	Examples	Occurrence
Needs to express symptoms, concerns, fears, interests, desire for information, and other ideas[a]	Worry about cancer Sore throat Feeling down Desire to lose weight Fever Refill medications	Very common
Special communication needs[b]	Deafness Blindness Muteness Cognitive deficit	Common
Urgent, sometimes life-threatening needs requiring immediate attention[c]		
Medical	Loss of consciousness Hematemesis Symptoms of acute myocardial infarction Recent history of syncope Severe pain Severe nausea and vomiting Marked shortness of breath	Uncommon
Psychosocial	Suicidal or homicidal ideation Disruptiveness Overt psychosis Severe organic brain syndrome Agitation or extreme anxiety	Uncommon

[a]Addressed in Chapters 1–5.
[b]Addressed in Chapter 6.
[c]Not addressed in this book.

urgent disease problem that dictates immediate doctor-directed input; for example, loss of consciousness, acute chest pain, profound shortness of breath, overt disruptiveness, extreme anxiety, or active psychosis. If one of these features is present, the interviewer takes charge and acts immediately to address the problem. In these unusual and generally obvious circumstances, the patient needs the interviewer to direct the process.

The vast majority of patients, however, have no such threatening problem, are able to communicate, are not prohibitively anxious, and want to talk about their symptoms, interests, fears, and concerns. In these more common situations, the interviewer initially meets the patient's needs, not by taking control but by allowing the patient to lead the conversation and to discuss the symptoms or personal issues she prefers. Ideas in the initial dialogue originate in the patient's mind rather than in the doctor's; later, the doctor will insert her ideas into the exchange.

I will address the common circumstance first, in Chapters 2 through 5, and will consider the interviewing approach to communication problems in Chapter 6; the approach to emergency medical and psychological conditions will be considered elsewhere in clinical training.

The Rationale for Integrated Patient-Doctor Interviewing

Most students recognize that a powerful humanistic rationale exists for integrating patient-centered principles and first addressing patients' needs. We then hear and understand our patients in a way that validates them as human beings rather than as objects of study [30]. As we strengthen our patients' involvement, sense of self-sufficiency, and feeling of responsibility, they are more likely to share power with the doctor and to feel autonomous [31]. Thus, effective communication involves a patient who is the expert on her or his needs and a doctor who is the expert at translating these needs into diagnoses of disease and treatment [9,10,31]. Physicians and students likewise benefit. They can fully express such human attributes as respect, empathy, humility, and sensitivity. Because these qualities seem less valued in the isolated doctor-centered approach, physicians have long felt guilty in expressing them, often surreptitiously employing them and even admonishing colleagues to "not tell anyone." The ideal of developing a feeling of connectedness between doctor and patient can become reality with a patient-centered approach, at times allowing previously unexperienced dimensions of caring, love, and spirituality to enter [32]. Both doctor and patient feel better [32–34].

A large body of evidence shows the deficiencies of an isolated doctor-centered approach. For example, one study showed that physicians did not allow patients to complete their opening statement of symptoms and concerns in 69 percent of visits, interrupting patients after a mean time of 18 seconds [35]. Information was obtained almost entirely through doctor-centered inquiry. Another study found that doctor-centered interviewing uncovered only 6 percent of the primary problems that were ultimately determined to be psychosocial [36]. Still another study found that an incomplete database was occasioned by omitting personal information and using a "high control" style [37]. These studies show that much patient data are physician determined, skewed toward physical symptoms and directed away from the personal dimension and the patient's concerns [22].

Numerous studies support the superiority of patient-centered approaches. Patient-centered interviewing produces personal data and emotional material [38–40]; much of the symptom data ordinarily obtained via doctor-centered inquiry [6]; and some physical symptom information not elicited by doctor-centered approaches, often of great value for diagnosing organic diseases [41].

Studies show increased patient satisfaction when patient-centered approaches are included, in contrast to isolated doctor-centered approaches [33,34,42]. This satisfaction, in turn, may decrease malpractice suits [43,44] and "doctor shopping" [45]. Patient-centered approaches enhance patient compliance [21,34,42] and increase the patient's knowledge and recall [33,34,42]. Improved recall, satisfaction, and compliance are, in turn, closely linked to better health status outcomes. For example, patient-centered approaches produce better blood pressure and diabetic control [46], improved perinatal outcome [47], and shortened and less complicated postoperative courses [48].

Inevitably, these data raise the question of how scientific a doctor-centered approach is. I believe that an isolated doctor-centered approach is at odds with scientific requirements, producing not only incomplete but biased data about the patient. An integrated approach demonstrably produces more complete and more valid data about the patient—who is, after all, the subject of the science of medicine [9,15,35–37,49,50]. No studies have compared the consistency of data obtained by the old and new approaches [9]. Theoretically, patient-centered data should be more consistent and less biased because they are far less influenced by the interviewer.

An additional attribute of a patient-centered approach, the student will be relieved to learn, is that it quickly elicits both personal and symptom data that are highly relevant for developing a biopsychosocial description of the patient [9]. In fact, these data efficiently point to the most important problem the patient has at a given time [9].

Integrated Patient-Doctor Interviewing

The patient-centered process of Integrated Patient-Doctor Interviewing precedes an often longer doctor-centered process [9]. We discourage interviewers from starting with the doctor-centered process. Even if they later introduce the patient-centered process, this order would suggest that the doctor's agenda is more important, an error except in the rare emergency situations noted earlier. When, later, a doctor-centered style predominates, the interviewer may return to a patient-centered process and frequently may need to move back and forth between the two processes. The student maintains a patient-centered attitude throughout the interview, supports the patient, and remains aware of the patient's needs.

Integrated Patient-Doctor Interviewing is the basis for most interactions: new or return patients, ward setting or clinic, surgery or medicine, tertiary care or primary care, emergency room or consultation visit. One determines the specific amount of time to be spent with the opening, patient-centered process by the extent and urgency of an individual patient's personal issues.

Integrated Patient-Doctor Interviewing describes the process of interviewing. The content it generates is usually obtained in this order with a new patient [51–60]: chief complaint (CC), history of present illness (HPI), other current active problems (OCAP), health issues (HI), past medical history (PMH), social history (SH), family history (FH), and review of systems (ROS). This content is later synthesized and condensed into the biopsychosocial description of the patient. In already known patients, we may need only the CC and HPI because other data are available from previous visits. The CC is the patient's most bothersome complaint, a part of their agenda. The HPI is usually the most helpful historical component where the patient gives both physical symptoms of possible disease and the personal context in which they occur. Most patients have more than one current medical concern, however, and the interviewer obtains these in OCAP. In HI, the interviewer inquires about relevant ethical-social-spiritual issues, functional capacity, health-promoting behaviors, and health hazards. In the PMH, the patient gives important past information not germane to the HPI or OCAP. In the SH, the patient provides routine personal data not already obtained as relevant and the FH does the same with routine family data. Of lowest priority, in the ROS, the student screens for any physical symptoms or other problems not already discussed. Ordinarily the CC/HPI/OCAP takes approximately half the total time available. The CC and initial portions of HPI/OCAP are developed using a patient-centered process while the latter portions of the HPI/OCAP develop using a doctor-centered process. The HI, PMH, FH, SH, and ROS develop largely by using a doctor-centered process.

With this process and content of the interview, it is logical to ask about its intended function or outcome. Recent major contributions by Bird, Cohen-Cole, and Lazare identify three distinct functions: (1) data-gathering, (2) establishing a relationship with the patient, and (3) patient education [61–63]. Some physicians see data-gathering, the act of obtaining relevant information about the patient, as the only function of the interview. Equally important are relationship-building, which deals with emotional issues, and patient education, which provides the patient with necessary information and motivates the patient to action when required.

Having identified the general interviewing process, its content, and expected functions, we still are left with an unanswered question: What actually goes on in the clinic or at the bedside? We are now ready to address what we do to elicit the patient's story and how we do it.

References

1. Engel GL. White coats, intimacy, and medicine as a human science. Presented at The Program for Biopsychosocial Studies, The University of Rochester School of Medicine and Dentistry; Rochester, NY; June 3, 1994.
2. Simpson M, et al. Doctor-patient communication: The Toronto consensus statement. *Br Med J* 303:1385–1387, 1991.
3. Peterson MC, et al. Contributions of the history, physical examination, and laboratory investigation in making medical diagnoses. *West J Med* 156:163–165, 1992.
4. Schmitt BP, Kushner MS, Wiener SL. The diagnostic usefulness of the history of the patient with dyspnea. *J Gen Intern Med* 1:386–393, 1986.
5. Hampton JR, et al. Relative contributions of history-taking, physical examination, and laboratory investigation to diagnosis and management of medical outpatients. *Brit Med J* 2:486–489, 1975.
6. Linfors EW, Neelon FA. Interrogation and interview: strategies for obtaining clinical data. *J R Coll Gen Pract [Occas Pap]* 31:426–428, 1981.
7. Lipkin M. The medical interview as core clnical skill: the problem and the opportunity. *J Gen Intern Med* 2:363–365, 1987.

8. Stoeckle JD, Billings A. A history of history-taking: the medical interview. *J Gen Intern Med* 2:119–127, 1987.
9. Smith RC, Hoppe RB. The patient's story: Integrating the patient- and physician-centered approaches to interviewing. *Ann Intern Med* 115:470–477, 1991.
10. Watzlawick P, Bavelas JB, Jackson DD. *Pragmatics of Human Communication: A Study of Interactional Patterns, Pathologies, and Paradoxes*. New York: WW Norton, 1967.
11. Foss L, Rothenberg K. *The Second Medical Revolution: From Biomedicine to Infomedicine*. Boston: Shambhala, 1987.
12. Lipkin M. Foreword. In *The Medical Interview: The Three Function Approach*. St. Louis, MO: Mosby-Year Book, 1991. Pp. vii–x.
13. Bean RB, Bean WB (eds.). *Sir William Osler Aphorisms: From His Bedside Teachings and Writings*. Springfield, IL: Charles C. Thomas, 1961.
14. Schwartz MA, Wiggins O. Science, humanism, and the nature of medical practice: a phenomenological view. *Perspect Biol Med* 28:331–361, 1985.
15. Feinstein AR. The intellectual crisis in clinical science: medaled models and muddled mettle. *Perspect Biol Med* 30:215–230, 1987.
16. Engel GL. The clinical application of the biopsychosocial model. *Am J Psychiatry* 137:535–544, 1980.
17. Engel GL. The need for a new medical model: a challenge for biomedicine. *Science* 196:129–136, 1977.
18. von Bertalanffy L. *General System Theory: Foundations, Development, Application*. Revised ed. New York, NY: George Braziller, 1968.
19. Weiss PA. *The Science of Life: The Living System—A System for Living*. Mount Kisco, NY: Futura, 1973.
20. Brody H. The systems view of man: implications for medicine, science, and ethics. *Perspect Biol Med* 17:71–92, 1973.
21. Lazare A. Hidden conceptual models in clinical psychiatry. *N Engl J Med* 288:345–351, 1973.
22. Waitzkin H. *The Politics of Medical Encounters: How Patients and Doctors Deal with Social Problems*. New Haven, Connecticut: Yale University Press, 1991.
23. Levenstein JH, et al. The patient-centered clinical method. 1. A model for the doctor-patient interaction in family medicine. *J Fam Pract* 3:24–30, 1986.
24. McWhinney I. The Need for a Transformed Clinical Method. In Stewart M, Roter D (eds.), *Communicating with Medical Patients*. London: Sage Publications, 1989. Pp. 25–42.
25. Levenstein JH, et al. Patient Centered Clinical Interviewing. In Stewart M, Roter D (eds.), *Communicating with Medical Patients*. London: Sage Publications, 1989. Pp. 107–120.
26. McWhinney I. *An Introduction to Family Medicine*. New York: Oxford University Press, 1981.

27. Rogers CR. *Client-Centered Therapy*. Boston: Houghton Mifflin, 1951.
28. Engel GL, et al. A graduate and undergraduate teaching program on the psychological aspects of medicine: A report on the liaison program between medicine and psychiatry at the University of Rochester School of Medicine. *J Med Educ* 32:859–871, 1957.
29. Tresolini CP, Pew-Fetzer Task Force. *Health Professions Education and Relationship-Centered Care*. San Francisco: Pew Health Professions Commission, 1994.
30. Mishler EG. *The Discourse of Medicine*. Norwood, NJ: Ablex Publishing Corp., 1984.
31. Brody H. *The Healer's Power*. New Haven: Yale University Press, 1992.
32. Suchman AL, Matthews DA. What makes the patient-doctor relationship therapeutic? Exploring the connexional dimension of medical care. *Ann Intern Med* 108:125–130, 1988.
33. Roter DL, Hall JA, Katz NR. Relations between physicians' behaviors and analogue patients' satisfaction, recall, and impressions. *Med Care* 25:437–451, 1987.
34. Hall JA, Roter DL, Katz NR. Meta-analysis of correlates of provider behavior in medical encounters. *Med Care* 26:657–675, 1988.
35. Beckman HB, Frankel RM. The effect of physician behavior on the collection of data. *Ann Intern Med* 101:692–696, 1984.
36. Burack RC, Carpenter RR. The predictive value of the presenting complaint. *J Fam Pract* 16:749–754, 1983.
37. Platt FW, McMath JC. Clinical hypocompetence: the interview. *Ann Intern Med* 91:898–902, 1979.
38. Cox A, Holbrook D, Rutter M. Psychiatric Interviewing techniques VI. Experimental study: eliciting feelings. *Br J Psychiatry* 139:144–152, 1981.
39. Hopkinson K, Cox A, Rutter M. Psychiatric interviewing techniques III. Naturalistic study: eliciting feelings. *Br J Psychiatry* 138:406–415, 1981.
40. Cox A, Rutter M, Holbrook D. Psychiatric interviewing techniques—a second experimental study: eliciting feelings. *Br J Psychiatry* 152:64–72, 1988.
41. Cox A, Rutter M, Holbrook D. Psychiatric interviewing techniques V. Experimental study: eliciting factual information. *Br J Psychiatry* 139:29–37, 1981.
42. Roter D. Which Facets of Communicaiton Have Strong Effects on Outcome—a Metaanalysis. In Stewart M, Roter D (eds.), *Communicating with Medical Patients*. London: Sage Publications, 1989. Pp. 183–196.
43. Vacarinno JM. Malpractice—the problem in perspective. *JAMA* 238:861–863, 1977.
44. Huycke LI, Huycke MM. Characteristics of potential plaintiffs in malpractice litigation. *Ann Intern Med* 120:792–798, 1994.
45. Kasteler J, et al. Issues underlying prevalence of "doctor-shopping" behavior. *J Health Soc Behav* 17:328–339, 1976.

46. Kaplan SH, Greenfield S, Ware JE. Impact of the Doctor-Patient Relationship on the Outcomes of Chronic Disease. In Stewart M, Roter D (eds.), *Communicating with Medical Patients*. London: Sage Publications, 1989. Pp. 228–245.

47. Shear CL, et al. Provider continuity and quality of medical care—a retrospective analysis of prenatal and perinatal outcome. *Med Care* 21:1204–1210, 1983.

48. Egbert LD, et al. Reduction of postoperative pain by encouragement and instruction of patients—a study of doctor-patient rapport. *N Engl J Med* 270:825–827, 1964.

49. Feinstein AR. An additional basic science for clinical medicine: I. The constraining fundamental paradigms. *Ann Intern Med* 99: 393–397, 1983.

50. Odegaard CE. *Dear Doctor: A Personal Letter to a Physician*. Menlo Park, CA: Henry J. Kaiser Family Foundation, 1986.

51. Morgan WL, Engel GL. *The Clinical Approach to the Patient*. Philadelphia: Saunders, 1969.

52. Reiser DE, Schroder AK. *Patient Interviewing—The Human Dimension*. Baltimore: Williams & Wilkins, 1980.

53. Cassel EJ. *Talking with Patients* (vols. 1 and 2). Cambridge: The MIT Press, 1985.

54. Billings AJ, Stoeckle JD. *The Clinical Encounter—A Guide to the Medical Interview and Case Presentation*. Chicago: Year Book, 1989.

55. Enelow AJ, Swisher SN. *Interviewing and Patient Care*. New York: Oxford University Press, 1986.

56. Coulehan JL, Block MR. *The Medical Interview: A Primer for Students of The Art*. Philadelphia: F. A. Davis, 1987.

57. Cohen-Cole SA. *The Medical Interview: The Three Function Approach*. St. Louis: Mosby–Year Book, 1991.

58. Greenspan SI, Greenspan NT. *The Clinical Interview of the Child* (2nd ed.). Washington, DC: American Psychiatric Press, 1991.

59. Levinson D. *A Guide to the Clinical Interview*. Philadelphia: Saunders, 1987.

60. Platt FW. *Conversation Repair*. Boston: Little, Brown, 1995.

61. Bird J, Cohen-Cole SA. The Three-Function Model of the Medical Interview: An Educational Device. In Hale M (ed.), *Models of Teaching Consultation-Liaison Psychiatry*. Basel: Karger, 1991. Pp. 65–88.

62. Cohen-Cole SA, Bird J. Interviewing the cardiac patient: II. A practical guide for helping patients cope with their emotions. *Quality of Life and Cardiovasc Care* 3:53–65, 1986.

63. Lazare A, Putnam S, Lipkin M. Three Functions of the Medical Interview. In Lipkin M, Putnam S, Lazare A (eds.), *The Medical Interview*. New York: Springer-Verlag, 1995. Pp. 3–19.

2

Facilitating Skills

Facilitating skills are the machinery of Integrated Patient-Doctor Interviewing. I will present them in detail in this chapter. Once learned, their synthesis during Integrated Patient-Doctor Interviewing, presented in Chapters 3 and 5, will fall into place easily. There are two categories of Facilitating Skills: Questioning Skills and Relationship-Building Skills, as summarized in Table 2-1. The skills in these two categories are the interviewer's tools on a moment-to-moment basis during the interview.

Questioning Skills

Open-Ended Skills
Open-ended questions are those that do not encourage yes or no answers or short answers. These questions elicit the patient's description, in the patient's own words, of symptoms and personal concerns. Open-ended inquiry usually provides information from the patient's mind, rather than from the interviewer's. Used repeatedly, open-ended skills can generate a story reflecting just the patient.

The six skills (see Table 2-1) are silence, nonverbal encouragement, neutral utterances, reflection, requests, and summarizing. The first three "nonfocusing" skills encourage the patient to talk but are not useful in focusing on a particular topic. These are familiar, easily learned, and used primarily during initial portions of the patient-centered process. The last three "focusing" skills, on the other hand, not only encourage the patient to talk but also focus talk on a particular topic. These more active patient-centered skills focus the patient during much of the patient-centered process of the interview.

Table 2-1. Facilitating skills

1. Questioning skills
   a. Open-ended
      (1) Silence[a]
      (2) Nonverbal encouragement[a]
      (3) Neutral utterances, continuers[a]
      (4) Reflection, echoing[b]
      (5) Open-ended requests[b]
      (6) Summary, paraphrasing[b]
   b. Closed-ended
      (1) Yes or no answers
      (2) Brief answers
2. Relationship-building skills
   a. Emotion-seeking
      (1) Direct
      (2) Indirect: self-disclosure, impact on life, impact on others, and belief about problem
   b. Emotion-handling
      (1) Naming, labeling
      (2) Understanding, legitimation
      (3) Respecting, praising
      (4) Supporting, partnership

[a]Nonfocusing open-ended skills.
[b]Focusing open-ended skills.
Adapted from Morgan WL, Engel GL. *The Clinical Approach to the Patient*. Philadelphia: Saunders, 1969 and Cohen-Cole SA. *The Medical Interview: The Three-Function Approach*. St. Louis: Mosby–Year Book, 1991.

Silence

Saying nothing while continuing to be attentive signals that the interviewer is listening. Silence prompts the patient to fill the space.

> **PT:**   . . . and it rolled down and hit me here . . . (pause)
> **DOC:**   (attentive but silent for 7 seconds)
> **PT:**   . . . so I called you, thinking you'd be in, but then . . .

But sometimes silence can make the patient uncomfortable, a discomfort he may indicate by shifting about or looking away. If 5 to 10 seconds of silence does not prompt further information, the interviewer uses another skill, especially if the patient seems uncomfortable.

Nonverbal Encouragement

Nonverbal encouragement urges patients to talk, is common-place in everyday interactions, and is much easier to use than silence. Typically, the interviewer gestures with the hand (rotatory motion to continue), makes a sympathetic facial expression (of expectation to continue), or simply indicates by body language that the patient should continue speaking (leaning forward).

PT: . . . so that it hurt his feelings (pause)
DOC: (leans forward with expectant expression on face)
PT: Well then I felt bad too and . . .

Neutral Utterances, Continuers

Neutral utterances encourage patients to continue talking and are another example of open-ended skills we use all the time, particularly in conjunction with nonverbal responses. These are nothing more than brief, noncommital statements such as "Oh," "Uh-huh," "Yes," or "Mmm."

PT: . . . and later the pain went in the front part, right here . . .
DOC: Uh-huh.
PT: Yeah, and it hurt like crazy.
DOC: Mmm.

Reflection, Echoing

Reflection (or echoing) states what the patient has just said, using the same word or phrase. Reflection signals that the interviewer has heard what was said and encourages the patient to proceed, especially focusing the patient on the word or phrase echoed.

PT: After the pain let up, I still couldn't find him.
DOC: The pain? (will focus patient on symptom of pain) —or—
Couldn't find him? (will focus patient on personal aspects)

Open-Ended Requests

Open-ended requests can be as general as "Tell me more" or "Go on." They also can be quite specific in focusing the patient in an already mentioned area that the interviewer wants to expand upon, such as "Tell me more about the daughter you mentioned." These directions move patients to deeper levels of their stories.

PT: Then my pain came back because I couldn't afford the medicine.

DOC: Go on (encourages patient to continue without focusing). — *or* — Tell me about not affording it (focuses patient on the personal problem). — *or* — Tell me about the pain (focuses patient on physical problem).

Summary, Paraphrasing

Instead of echoing only a word or phrase, the interviewer echoes a wider range of talk by summarizing it. Summarizing focuses patients on the material summarized and prompts them to express deeper levels of their stories. It signals that they have been heard and encourages them to proceed beyond that point.

PT: (long story about difficulty getting in to see doctor)

DOC: So you had the nausea but couldn't get me on the phone. Then it got worse and your wife still couldn't get ahold of me until today.

PT: Yeah, I was really more upset than sick by now.

Closed-Ended Skills

Closed-ended questions are answerable by yes or no or by a brief response. They usually are used to focus on specific issues in the interviewer's mind. This makes them ideal for the doctor-centered process in which many details have to be obtained and the interviewer takes the lead. Closed-ended questions enhance the precision of information. Used alone, however, they are counterproductive. They discourage information originating in the patient's mind and force the patient to the doctor's concerns and ideas. Used in isolation, closed-ended skills also can have a deleterious effect upon the doctor-patient relationship, can greatly diminish the quantity and quality of data about the patient, and are inefficient.

There are two types of closed-ended skills (see Table 2-1), both very familiar and reflexive.

Questions Producing Yes or No Answers

These questions are asked with a specific issue to be answered.

PT: My pain is right here.

DOC: Is there any shortness of breath? — *or* — Does it go out your arm? — *or* — Did your wife come with you?

PT: No.

DOC: Did you come in this morning?
PT: Yes.

Questions Producing Brief Answers
These questions are similar in type and function.

DOC: How old are you?
PT: 31.
DOC: How high was the fever?
PT: I don't know. — or — 103 degrees.

Integrating Open-Ended and Closed-Ended Skills
Open-ended and closed-ended skills complement each other. During the patient-centered process, open-ended questions predominate and are used repeatedly, primarily for developing personal data about symptoms and other concerns. Closed-ended questions are much less prominent and are used for clarifying purposes. During the doctor-centered process, open-ended questions may be fewer and used primarily for brief but repeated scanning purposes, the bulk of the work being done more effectively with closed-ended questions to pin down details.

Relationship-Building Skills

Relationship-building skills elicit and then address the patient's emotions. Expressing needs through emotion antedates language and is a basic form of human communication [1–3]. Not surprisingly, addressing emotion leads to development of the strongest possible doctor-patient relationship and is the quickest route to elicit data reflecting the patient's personal life [2,4]. Because of the centrality of emotion to human function [1–7], understanding the patient's emotional life often takes precedence over understanding other aspects of the patient's life. As described later, the student will learn that one does not use these skills until the patient feels comfortable and knows that the interviewing circumstance is a safe setting for addressing emotions.

Emotions can be expressed in three ways: (1) acting them out (crying), (2) nonverbal expression (depressed faces, slumped shoulders), and (3) verbal statements ("I was upset"). Many different emotional states are listed in Appendix A to give the student an idea of what constitutes emotion and how vast this area is; most students are surprised to learn how many different emotions there are.

Emotion-Seeking Skills

Because emotions are so important, I recommend that students actively seek them even when they are not presented—or when only partially expressed. The emotion-seeking skills serve this purpose. Once emotions are clearly present and fully developed, the interviewer employs the subsequently described emotion-handling skills.

The student uses the following methods to seek emotion, often starting in the order given below but subsequently interspersing them freely. Typically, direct inquiry suffices to elicit the initial emotion and indirect inquiry further develops it. In more reticent patients, indirect inquiry is sometimes required to initiate expression.

Direct Inquiry

One of the most important questions in interviewing is some variation of "How did that make you feel?" Directly asking does not mean inserting the hypothesized feeling ("Did you feel angry?") but letting the patient identify the specific feeling. The interviewer asks this question when emotion is suspected from the patient's statement ("she got my job"), from nonverbal behavior (shifts in chair), or when the patient shows no reaction in a situation where emotion is likely (death of spouse). Most respond to this invitation. Some patients may not understand and respond with how they feel physically ("sick to my stomach"). The interviewer circumvents this by asking "How did you feel emotionally, personally?"

> **PT:**   (has just mentioned his wife is leaving)
> **DOC:**   So, how's that make you feel, you know, personally?
> **PT:**   Surprised, I guess (but looking sad).
> **DOC:**   How are you feeling right now, talking about it?

When patients already are expressing emotion and its nature is obvious (crying after loss of spouse), one does not inquire specifically about the feeling but often will inquire to further develop it, such as "I can see you're very sad, can you tell me more about what it's like for you?"

Indirect Inquiry

Emotional expression does not always follow direct inquiry. Because emotions are so important, however, one continues seeking them. There are four ways, not necessarily used in this order, in which the student encourages the reticent patient or further develops already expressed emotion.

1. Self-disclosure may help ("I once had a similar experience and I was very upset"). One avoids loaded emotional terms *(anger, depressed)* and uses more neutral terms for emotions such as *upset, unhappy,* or *frustrated.*
2. Inquiring about how the illness or other situation in question has affected the patient's life also uncovers important information and increases emotional expression ("Since your wife died, how's this affected your life?").
3. Inquiring about how the circumstance has affected others is a more subtle way to encourage emotional expression ("How's your wife's death affected your daughter?").
4. Inquiring about what the patient thinks is the cause or mechanism of the problem also elicits emotional expression ("Why do you think the cancer got worse?").

> **PT:** (patient has just been fired but acknowledges no emotion with direct inquiry)
>
> **DOC:** That happened to me once and I was upset. *– or –* How's it going to affect your life? *– or –* What will your wife say? *– or –* Why do you think you lost it?

Emotion-Handling Skills (Relationship-Building)

The aptly named emotion-handling skills manage or "handle" emotion, once expressed. These are essential in developing a positive doctor-patient relationship [8]. The mnemonic NURS helps recall them: Naming, Understanding, Respecting, and Supporting (i.e., one NURS(es) the emotion). We sometimes use all four skills in this precise order, as shown in the vignette, but more often one or two at a time is used.

Naming, Labeling the Emotion

The interviewer names the emotion identified; for example, "That sounds sad for you." As suggested above, the word *sad* connotes less emotion rather than more, such as using "frustrated" rather than "angry." Our message: The patient has been heard and the interviewer has properly recognized the emotion.

Understanding, Legitimation

The interviewer acknowledges that the emotional reaction is understandable; for example, "Given what happened it makes sense to me; I can sure understand why." The emotion is thus legitimized, accepted, and validated. The interviewer's statement must be genuine, which means both having heard enough about the story to satisfactorily understand it and also have sufficient experience with the particular issue to be able to understand it. Indeed, one can indicate lack of comparable experiences with equal impact in appropriate circumstances; for example, when the patient has just lost all members of her family in an automobile accident, the response might be "I've never had that happen, but I can see how deeply it hurts."

Respecting, Praising

Respecting and praising are the most difficult and least natural of the NURS quartet. Many interviewers already are behaving respectfully, via their nonverbal behaviors, and don't understand what else is needed. Verbal respecting statements clearly acknowledge how difficult things have been for the patient ("You've really been through a lot") or praise them for their efforts ("I like the way you've hung in there and kept fighting"). This often involves emphasizing the positive—finding what people have done well and reinforcing it. Again, one praises only after having sufficient data to legitimately do so.

Supporting, Partnership

The interviewer indicates that he, and perhaps others, are available for support and are "in the soup with you" to do whatever they can to help. Not only is one willing to help but is available to do it together as a team with the patient; for example, "I'm here to help in any way I can. Together, you and I, we can get to the bottom of this."

Brief Vignette Using NURS Quartet

PT: (has just indicated feeling lonely since his dog died)
DOC: So, that's been pretty lonesome for you. *[Naming]*
PT: We were together for a long time. Sounds kind of silly, I know.

DOC: Not at all. I had a dog die a couple years ago. I can really understand. We grieve all our losses — dogs as well as people. It makes sense to me. *[Understanding]*

PT: He always used to ride in the car with me.

DOC: He meant a lot to you. I can see it's been a difficult time. *[Respecting]*

PT: It really has.

DOC: Sometimes it helps talking about it. *[Supporting]*

PT: It does feel better. I was embarassed to mention it to anyone else.

The interviewer does not have to agree with the emotion for which she indicates understanding, respect, or support. Rather, she is indicating appreciation of the patient's point of view and circumstance. To an abusive parent one might say "I understand how all her crying upset you," or "It's really been hard on you," or "I'm here to help you do what's best" — without condoning or reinforcing abusive behavior.

Addressing emotions provokes anxiety in some interviewers, for example, the fear of harming a patient. This common fear is groundless and, indeed, the truth is quite the opposite. Another fear of some interviewers is that emotional expression will get out of control. Patients, however, easily control how far they want to go and the interviewer always controls how far she wants to proceed. Thus, patients can be allowed and encouraged to express emotion. Interviewers must guard against the understandable impulse to shut them off or change the subject. Many find this a difficult new area.

Patient-Centered and Doctor-Centered Interviewing Further Defined

I now specify how we use the just-described skills in a patient-centered or doctor-centered approach. Patient-centered interviewing means addressing open-ended skills, emotion-seeking skills, and emotion-handling skills to material *already introduced* by the patient. Indeed, with many of these skills, one cannot do otherwise; for example, neutral utterances, echoing, summarizing, naming, and understanding can be applied only after the patient introduces the material to which they are addressed. By focusing on material already introduced, these skills encourage the patient's lead. The interviewer, however, can refocus the patient on an important topic that may have slipped by too quickly. Often patients mention a loaded topic, such as death, but rapidly move away from it. The interviewer can return to the topic by saying, for example, "You mentioned death a minute ago, tell me more about that." Because the patient initially introduced the topic of death, this action is patient-centered even though interrupting the immediate thread of conversation. On the other hand, to be most patient-centered, one avoids shifting away from important personal topics back to physical symptoms already mentioned. By applying these skills to material already introduced by the patient, the interviewer obtains a story that originates more completely from the patient's mind, and is less "contaminated" by the interviewer's thoughts and actions. To be certain, the interviewer always will influence and have an effect upon the conversation, but a patient-centered approach minimizes the impact and precludes the gross contamination of conversation that occurs, with a doctor-centered approach.

Open-ended requests (one of the focusing open-ended skills) and emotion-seeking skills, in addition to closed-ended skills, also can be used to focus on a topic not yet introduced by the patient. Such action is not patient-centered; for example, when "health" or "wife" have not been mentioned or alluded to by the patient, it would not be patient-centered to say "Tell me about your health" (an open-ended request) or "What are your feelings about your wife?" (direct emotion-seeking). *Inquiry that introduces new information contaminates the conversation with the interviewer's ideas and is, by definition, doctor-centered;* that is, the doctor is determining the direction and content of conversation. Such inquiry is appropriate during the doctor-centered process where one frequently must introduce ideas and concepts not yet mentioned by the patient — using open-ended requests (frequently), emotion-seeking skills (rarely), and, primarily, closed-ended skills.

Summary

The facilitating skills described in this chapter are the tools for implementing Integrated Patient-Doctor Interviewing. As fully described in Chapters 3 and 5, they are integrated in both patient-centered and doctor-centered processes but are used in different balances and for different purposes. The relationship-building skills, because of their close link to the patient's emotional life, are the key elements in efficiently eliciting information and establishing a relationship. Open-ended skills, emotion-seeking skills, and emotion-handling skills are the tools for implementing a patient-centered approach, but they must be used in a way that does not introduce new data to the conversation. Some of these skills, open-ended requests and emotion-seeking skills, also can be used, along with closed-ended skills, in a doctor-centered approach where the interviewer does introduce new data and determine the direction and content of the conversation.

References

1. Engel GL. *Psychological Development in Health and Disease*. Philadelphia: Saunders, 1962.
2. Holmes J. Attachment theory: A biological basis for psychotherapy? *Br J Psychiatry* 163:430–438, 1993.
3. Damasio AR. *Descartes' Error*. New York: GP Putnam's Sons, 1994.
4. Smith RC, Hoppe RB. The patient's story: integrating the patient- and physician-centered approaches to interviewing. *Ann Intern Med* 115:470–477, 1991.
5. Fenichel O. *The Psychoanalytical Theory of Neurosis*. New York: WW Norton, 1945.
6. Brenner C. *An Elementary Textbook of Psychoanalysis* (revised ed.). Garden City, NY: Anchor Press/Doubleday, 1964.
7. Fancher RE. *Psychoanalytic Psychology: The Development of Freud's Thought*. New York: WW Norton, 1973.
8. Platt FW, Keller VF. Empathic communication. *J Gen Intern Med* 9:222–226, 1994.

3

Patient-Centered Process

This chapter describes and demonstrates exactly what the interviewer does, step by step, during the patient-centered process, the first part of Integrated Patient-Doctor Interviewing. There are five steps in the patient-centered process. They enhance the patient's lead and expression of what is most important. An ongoing interview with "Mrs. Jones" is introduced to illustrate each step; this and other examples are derived from real people and situations but are sufficiently masked to protect confidentiality. To begin, we first address some patient-centered skills not yet introduced: setting the stage for the interview (step 1) and determining the agenda (includes the chief complaint) for the interview (step 2).

Setting the Stage for the Interview (Step 1)

Step 1 skills are sometimes overlooked courtesies that ensure a patient-centered atmosphere. Table 3-1 lists these skills in their usual order of use at the first meeting with a patient; appropriate adjustments are made when the patient is already known to the interviewer. These rapport-building skills enhance the relationship and establish or reaffirm participants' identities [1–3].

Welcome the Patient
The patient must feel valued and welcome. Simple statements suffice, such as "Welcome to the clinic" or, in a hospital setting, "Sorry to see you're sick but glad you came to see us." This sets the proper tone for a patient-centered interaction. The interviewer always tries to shake hands with the patient altough this is sometimes not possible with very ill patients; in the latter instance, a friendly pat on the hand or arm is equally beneficial to the relationship. The interviewer can develop some important initial nonverbal

Table 3-1.   Setting the stage for the interview (step 1)

1. Welcome the patient
2. Use the patient's name
3. Introduce self and identify specific role
4. Ensure patient readiness and privacy
5. Remove barriers to communication
6. Ensure comfort and put the patient at ease

Adapted from Smith RC, Hoppe RB. The patient's story: integrating the patient- and physician-centered approaches to interviewing. *Ann Intern Med* 115:470–477, 1991.

impressions about the patient from the handshake; for example, a hearty handshake suggesting a confident person, a cold sweaty palm suggesting anxiety, and the feeble handshake of someone very ill.

Use the Patient's Name

This can be done quite efficiently, combining one courtesy with another, such as "It's Mrs. Garcia isn't it? Welcome to the clinic." The interviewer uses the patient's last name unless the patient volunteers the use of another name. If the patient has a difficult name, the interviewer may need to ask how to pronounce it.

Introduce Self and Identify Specific Role

Although first names are permissible, the student usually begins using her or his last name and also notes her or his official role with the patient. Introductions can be combined with other patient-centered gestures, for example saying, "How do you do Mrs. Garcia, I'm Mr. Burns, the medical student who will be part of the team looking after you"; the student also can use the term *student doctor* to designate himself. Occasionally at the beginning, but more often after the relationship has matured, a first-name relationship develops. The student or physician carefully matches identity terms and, thereby, avoids suggesting an unequal relationship. That is, both student and patient are on a last name basis or they are on a first name basis; for example, one does not say, "Hi George, I'm Dr. Smith" or "Welcome Mr. Brown, I'm Betty."

Introductions can be difficult. The student often feels torn between misrepresenting himself as a doctor and not wanting to appear inept by conveying perceived lack of expertise ("I'm not a real doctor"). Honestly portraying one's situation goes a long way toward developing the student's sense of professional identity, particularly as patients repeatedly accept the student's professional role [2]. In addition to noting that you are a student doctor, one might say, "I'm part of the team taking care of you. I'll be getting much of the information about you and will be (one of) your major contact person(s)." It is not necessary to apologize or otherwise denigrate oneself ("I'm just a student, thanks for letting me talk to you."). Nor should there be any question about the patient's acceptance of a student working with them: The preceptor should have established that with the patient beforehand. Students must understand and confidently convey that they are indeed a key part of the patient's care. The annals of medicine are replete with stories of students' contributions to care, as they are with stories of patients deferring to students' opinions; for example, when the resident or faculty makes a recommendation directly to the patient, the patient says, "I'll have to ask my doctor [the student]."

Ensure Patient Readiness and Privacy
Initially, especially in hospital settings and with very ill patients, the student ascertains if the time is convenient for the patient. Sometimes it is necessary to postpone the interview; for example, until after the patient has eaten dinner or relatives have departed, until the vomiting attending recent chemotherapy has abated. Severe pain, severe nausea, need for a medication, and a soiled bed, for example, are other physical problems that must be addressed before the patient is ready for an interview. Because outpatients generally are healthier and have scheduled visits, postponement is less of an issue with these patients. Nevertheless, the interviewer also monitors patients' circumstances for nonphysical, potentially interfering problems; for example, a patient may have lost his car keys in the waiting room, just received a disturbing telephone call, or be worried that the baby-sitter will have to leave before he gets home. With all patients it is important to determine if there are pressing needs that might require brief delay in the interview; for example, to use the bathroom, get a drink of water. These courtesies not only help the patient directly but enhance the patient's acceptance of the student as a caring professional. Once ready, there can be some obvious actions that will improve the patient's readiness and privacy, such as shutting a door or respectfully excusing a curious laboratory technician.

Remove Barriers to Communication
The interviewer may have to turn off a noisy air conditioner or television set, or make efforts requiring more insight, such as

recognizing that the patient hears best out of one ear or that he needs to be able to directly see the interviewer's mouth in order to lip-read. If there is any question, the interviewer would inquire, "Can you hear me and see me okay?". Strategies for addressing specific communication problems are outlined in Chapter 6.

Ensure Comfort and Put the Patient at Ease

The interviewer determines if anything at the immediate time is interfering with the patient's comfort. A question like, "Is that a comfortable chair (bed) for you?" or "Is the light bothering your eyes?" is essential. The interviewer must continue to monitor the patient's state as the interview proceeds. The task is to put the patient at ease, as much as possible. Attention to these problems not only helps the patient and allows their subsequent full attention but also bespeaks the interviewer's professionality.

Where there are no such interfering problems, the usual circumstance, it is appropriate to conduct a little light conversation to put the patient at ease, as the above discussions will have done for patients with some problem. The student may be ready to start but the patient often is not and still doesn't know much about the interviewer. This conversation should have a patient focus such as, "I hope you got your car parked okay with all the construction going on around here." With an inpatient, one might inquire about their care or the food. Whatever is appropriate to the patient's situation can be briefly discussed. Patients get used to talking and also learn what the student is like. A caring, friendly atmosphere is established.

Obtaining the Agenda (Chief Complaint and Other Current Concerns) (Step 2)

In step 2, just as in setting the stage for the interview, the student takes charge and focuses the patient on the agenda [1–3]. Although student-originated, the action is also patient-centered because it establishes a patient-centered atmosphere. This step is not as easy as step 1 and serious pitfalls arise if conducted improperly. The following four skills, summarized in Table 3-2, usually are performed in the order given.

Table 3-2. Chief complaint/agenda setting (step 2)

1. Indicate time available
2. Indicate own needs
3. Obtain list of all issues patient wants to discuss; e.g., specific symptoms, requests, expectations, understanding
4. Summarize and finalize the agenda; negotiate specifics if too many agenda items

Adapted from Smith RC, Hoppe RB. The patient's story: integrating the patient- and physician-centered approaches to interviewing. *Ann Intern Med* 115:470–477, 1991.

Indicate Time Available
While setting limits often is difficult for interviewers, they should begin by indicating how much time is available for the interaction. This lets the patient know whether he has 10 or 60 minutes and helps him gauge what and how much to say [4].

Indicate Own Needs
The interviewer also indicates her own professional demands, such as needing to ask many questions to get a full history and needing to perform a physical examination with a new patient, or needing to follow up on a recent cholesterol test in a return patient.

Obtain List of All Issues Patient Wants to Discuss
Most important, the interviewer must obtain a list of all issues the patient wants to discuss [5,6]. The interviewer can begin, for example, by covering the above two items and then starting this one; for example, "We've got about an hour today and I need to ask a lot of questions and do an examination. But, more important, I'd like to know what you wanted to cover."

The interviewer wants the patient to enumerate all problems so they won't arise at the end when time has run out [4,7]. The doctor and patient can prioritize if too many issues are raised for this visit and determine which is most important, not always the first one given [8]. Enumeration goes beyond just symptoms and includes the patient's requests (prescription for a sedative), expectations (get sick leave), and understanding about what the interaction is supposed to do (perform a treadmill test). Nor is it sufficient to ask once. Rather, the interviewer carefully probes for additional issues of concern, trying to learn what is most important and why the patient came at this particular time. The interviewer needs to ask "What else?" or "Anything else?" or "How did you hope I could help?" or "What would a good result from this visit today look like?" It is unusual that patients have just one issue, more likely there are three to five. Careful agenda-setting prevents the common patient complaint that they didn't get to talk about all concerns as well as the common physician complaint that the patient voiced his most serious concern at the end of the appointment.

Although I have discussed the content of agenda-setting, we must consider how to perform it. At this point, one wants a list. Indeed, the student avoids details of any particular problem until the list is complete. This can be difficult because patients often want to go right into details. The student must respectfully interrupt the patient and refocus on the list. It helps to hold up one's fingers prominently and count the problems identified. For example, while holding up one finger to signify the first problem given, the interviewer might say "Sorry to interrupt and we'll get back to the leg pain, but first I need to know if there is a second problem you'd like to talk about. I want to be certain we know what all your concerns are." One often has to do this several times, for patients give many problems but want to discuss each as it arises.

Only if the patient raised highly charged emotional material while setting the agenda would the interviewer encourage further discussion at that point (e.g., if the patient is acutely distraught about a recent death in the family or a recent diagnosis of cancer in oneself). Even in most emotionally charged situations, however, the agenda usually can be set and the emotional material delayed briefly.

Summarize and Finalize Agenda
Usually, it is possible to cover all problems, in which case these are simply summarized. This also is a good point to determine, if not already known, which complaint is most important, that is, identify the chief complaint. When too many issues have been raised for just one visit, patient and interviewer negotiate and agree on what will be addressed and when the deferred issues will be considered. We now begin to follow Mrs. Joanne Jones through her initial visit by providing a continuous transcript for each step; some areas are shortened as noted for space considerations.

Vignette of Mrs. Jones
DOC: (enters examining room and shakes hands) Welcome to the clinic, Mrs Jones, I'm Mr. White, the medical student who will be working with you along with Dr. Black. I'll be getting much of the information about you and will be in close contact

with you about our findings and your subsequent care. *[Student welcomes the patient, uses her name, and identifies self and role]*

PT: Hi. I wasn't sure who I was going to see. This is my first time here.

DOC: If it's okay with you, I'll close this door so we can hear each other better and have some privacy. *[Student ensures readiness for the interview and establishes as much privacy as possible.]*

PT: Sure, that's fine.

DOC: Anything I can help with before we get started?

PT: Well, they didn't give my registration card back to me. I don't want to lose it.

DOC: We'll give that back when we're finished today. They always keep them. Anything else?

PT: No.

DOC: You may want to sit in that chair. It's more comfortable than the examining table. *[Student has noticed no barriers to communication and now ensures comfort and puts the patient at ease]*

PT: Sure. Thanks. (She moves)

DOC: Well, I'm glad to see you made it despite the snow. I thought spring was here last week.

PT: I guess not. My kids have been home the last two days. I'm ready to get them back to school! I'm getting spoiled with them both in school.

DOC: People have had all kinds of trouble getting in here for their appointments since the snow. It's no fun.

PT: You're telling me. I don't even ski! *[The student has set the stage, a light conversation has occurred, and the patient is joking.]*

DOC: (laughs) Well, we've got about an hour today and I know I've got a lot of questions to ask and that we need to do a physical exam. Before we get started, though, it's most important to find out what you wanted to cover today. You know, so we're sure everything gets covered. *[Student gives his agenda in one statement. Doing this first models the more difficult task to follow: obtaining the patient's agenda.]*

PT: It's these headaches. They start behind my eye and then I get sick to my stomach so I can't even work. My boss is really getting upset with me. He thinks that I don't have anything wrong with me and says he's going to report me. Well, he's not really my boss, but rather is . . . (student interrupts)

DOC: That sounds difficult and really important. Before we get into the details, though, I'd like to find out if there are any other problems you'd like to look at today, so we can cover everything you want to. We'll get back to the headache and your boss after that. That's two things (holding up two fingers). Is there anything else?

PT: Well, I wanted to find out about this cold that doesn't seem to go away. I've been coughing for 3 weeks.

DOC: (holding up three fingers now) Anything else you want to look at today?

PT: No. Well, I did want to find out if I need any medicine for my colitis. That's doing okay now but I've had real trouble in the past. My parents were very upset about that. It started bothering me way back in 1982 and I've had trouble off and on. I used to take cortisone and . . . (student interrupts) *[Student has now interrupted her twice in order to complete the list of complaints. This is necessary, done respectfully, to complete the agenda in a timely way.]*

DOC: (holding up five fingers) So there's two more problems we can look into, the colitis and the medications. We'll get back to all these soon. To make sure we get all your questons covered, though, is there anything else?

PT: No. The headache is the main thing.

DOC: So, we want to cover the headaches and the problem they cause at work, cough, colitis, and the medications for the colitis. Is that right? *[It is here that the patient and student would negotiate what to cover at this visit if the student determined that the patient had raised too many issues to cover on this day.]*

PT: That's about it.

DOC: And do I understand correctly that the headache is the worst problem? *[Mrs. Jones' headache is her most bothersome complaint, what we earlier defined as the chief complaint.]*

PT: Yes.

Beginning the History of the Present Illness (HPI): Nonfocused Interviewing (Step 3)

Having set the stage (step 1) and obtained the agenda (step 2), we now can incorporate the facilitating skills learned in Chapter 2

[1–3]. Step 3, summarized in Table 3-3, establishes an easy flow of talk from the patient, conveys that the doctor will listen, and gives a feel for "what the patient is like."

Open-Ended Beginning Question

Immediately after summarizing the agenda, the interviewer uses an open-ended beginning question such as, "Given what you've told me, how are you doing (. . . how are things going)?" One links the question to the agenda to start developing the story. When the patient has raised strong but deferred emotional material during agenda-setting, one can direct the patient back to it (e.g., "Now, you mentioned being upset?"). A good beginning question, befitting its nonfocusing intent, allows the patient to go anywhere, from the past to the present to the future, concerning anybody or anything.

Unless strong emotion has been expressed, the interviewer initially avoids framing the question in a way that specifies what the patient's problem is ("Now, what about the chest pain?" or "What about the trouble with your wife?"). Only if the patient continues to ask should the interviewer provide such instruction. To the query "What do you mean?" or "You mean about my chest pain?", the interviewer initially can reply "Whatever you like" or "Whatever is most important to you." The patient-centered intent is to allow free discussion but, at the same time, not to make patients uncomfortable or puzzled.

This open-ended beginning question is not always necessary. Having completed the agenda, especially if there is only one or a few related items, many patients continue spontaneously.

Table 3-3. Nonfocused interviewing (step 3)

1. Open-ended beginning question
2. Nonfocusing open-ended skills: silence, neutral utterances, nonverbal encouragement
3. Focusing open-ended inquiry also appropriate if needed to get patient talking: echoing, summary, requests
4. Closed-ended questions for clarification
5. Obtain additional data from the following sources: nonverbal cues, physical characteristics, autonomic changes, accoutrements, and environment

Adapted from Smith RC, Hoppe RB. The patient's story: integrating the patient- and physician-centered approaches to interviewing. *Ann Intern Med* 115:470–477, 1991.

Nonfocusing Open-Ended Skills
Following the open-ended beginning question, the student encourages a continued free flow of information, briefly using the nonfocusing open-ended skills. Silence, nonverbal gestures (eye contact, attentive behavior, hand gestures), and neutral utterances
("Uh-huh," "Mmm") encourage the patient. If the patient does not
talk freely, we can use the focusing open-ended skills (echoing,
request, summary) to promote a free flow of information; that is,
with a patient who is not talking, the interviewer should not
continue to just sit in silence and appear attentive. If focusing open-
ended skills are not effective, closed-ended questions about the
patient's problem may get a dialogue going. Whatever is needed to
get the patient talking is appropriate.

Although the interviewer is passive verbally during the brief
step 3, he is active mentally, thinking about what the information
means. One observes the patient for nonverbal cues, reviewed in
Chapter 7 (e.g., depressed faces, arms folded across chest, toes
tapping nervously). One also observes for clues in the following
areas that will give additional information about the patient
[9,10]:

1. Physical characteristics: general health, skin and hair color and
   odor, deformities, habitus (e.g., emaciated and disheveled,
   "uremic" breath, jaundice, amputated leg, kyphoscoliosis).
2. Autonomic changes: heart rate, skin color, pupil size, skin
   moisture, skin temperature (e.g., rapid pulsation of the carotid
   artery observed in the neck, handshake reveals cold and moist
   palms, pupils constricted but then dilate when relaxed, sweat-
   ing at outset of interview).
3. Accoutrements: clothing, jewelry, eyeglasses, make-up (e.g.,
   expensive suit and jewelry, thick eyeglasses, no make-up).
4. Environment: decorations, greeting cards, flowers, photogaphs
   (e.g., several paintings by a grandchild, photograph of spouse,
   no greeting cards or flowers—in a hospital setting).

Patients seldom show emotion in this early period but, if strong
emotion is expressed, one addresses it as explained in step 4.
Otherwise, the student simply observes where the patient is going
and how emotion fits with the rest of the evolving material. The
type of data being produced makes no difference. As long as a good
flow of information occurs, either symptoms (of possible disease)
or personal data are acceptable.

Continuation of Vignette of Mrs. Jones
(immediately continuous with the previous vignette)

PT: Yes.

DOC: So, that's a lot going on, how are you doing with it? *[A good open-ended beginning that is linked to the agenda allows the patient to go anywhere she wants.]*

PT: Oh, okay I guess.

DOC: (silence)

PT: At least now.

DOC: (sits forward slightly) Uh huh.

PT: Things weren't so good last week, though, when I made the appointment.

DOC: Mmmm.

PT: That's when my boss really got on me. Well, he's kind of uptight anyway, but he was saying how I was upsetting the whole office operation because I was off so much. And someone had to cover for me. I'm the lead attorney.

DOC: I see.

PT: These headaches are right here (points at right temple) and just throb and throb. And I get sick to my stomach and just don't feel good. All I want to do is go home and go to bed. *[A good open-ended beginning followed, briefly, by several nonfocusing open-ended skills have resulted in a good flow of symptoms and personal data without any focusing activity by the student.]*

Continuing the HPI: Focused Interviewing (Step 4)

The much longer step 4, summarized in Table 3-4, follows immediately. The intent changes from establishing a flow of information to, in addition, focusing on the most important theme(s) [1–3]. Themes usually involve a personal description of the physical symptoms and the more general personal concerns and emotions that attend the physical symptoms.

We use the focusing open-ended skills, emotion-seeking skills, and emotion-handling skills outlined in Chapter 2 to identify the theme(s) and, occasionally, closed-ended skills for clarification. The interviewer is much more active and participatory, often figuratively on the edge of the seat during the give-and-take interaction with the patient. The new interviewer may find this step the most difficult of

Table 3-4. Focused interviewing (step 4)

1. Obtain personal description of the symptoms [*focusing open-ended skills*]
2. Extend the personal story to the broader context of the symptoms [*focusing open-ended skills*]
3. Continue to develop a free flow of personal data [*focusing open-ended skills*]
4. Develop an emotional focus [*emotion-seeking skills*]
5. Address the emotion(s) [*emotion-handling skills*]
6. Use the "core dynamic skills" (focused open-ended skills, emotion-seeking skills, emotion-handling skills) to better identify and deepen the story
7. Conclude and address other current issues

Adapted from Smith RC, Hoppe RB. The patient's story: integrating the patient- and physician-centered approaches to interviewing. *Ann Intern Med* 115:470–477, 1991.

the entire interview. To aid understanding, I have broken it down into several segments, now considered in their usual sequence.

Obtain a Personal Description of the Symptoms
In a medical setting, patients typically present physical symptoms mixed with their personal context. The student first open-endedly focuses on the symptoms, using *focusing open-ended skills* (echoing, open-ended requests, summarizing). This produces a description in the patient's own words and the uniquely personal context in which the physical symptom occurred. Let's pick up Mrs. Jones' interview again.

Continuation of Vignette of Mrs. Jones

PT: . . . All I want to do is go home and go to bed.

DOC: Say more about the headaches. *[An open-ended request, one of the focusing open-ended skills. The student wants to know how the boss (personal data) and the headaches (symptoms) go together. To do this requires active focusing on material the patient introduces. Because her major complaint is headache, the interviewer starts with this, although could have continued by focusing on her boss]*

PT: Well, I never had any trouble until I got here. *[Comment about present personal context of her symptom]*

DOC: How long's that been? *[Appropriate closed-ended question for clarification]*

PT: Only 4 months. The headache started about 3 months ago.

DOC: You mentioned your boss. *[Echoing, another focusing open-ended skill, focuses the patient. Student is trying to see how the boss fits into this picture.]*

PT: It seems like every time I see him anymore I get one of these headaches. I sometimes just get a little nauseated but, if he's around much, there's the headache. *[Student learns much more of the immediate personal context of the symptom, data that cannot be obtained by closed-ended interviewing.]*

DOC: Keep going. *[A focusing open-ended request keeps the focus on her boss.]*

PT: Well, I have no trouble at all when he's not there. He was gone for 2 weeks and I didn't have any. But he's there a lot, although I don't have to be around him all the time. *[The relationship of Mrs. Jones' headaches and her boss are becoming clear.]*

DOC: Not around him? *[Echoing, a focusing open-ended skill, maintains the focus.]*

PT: I'm on the road a lot. No trouble then either, I guess. Except once when he called me. *[The headaches clearly relate to the presence of Mrs. Jones' boss. In less than a minute, the student has established the immediate personal context of the symptom, and how the personal and physical interact, by facilitating (encouraging) the patient's spontaneous narration. The personal description of the pain in this vignette has considerable diagnostic value (for migraine headaches) and also raises some considerations for treatment; e.g., avoiding her boss. Such unique data simply do not arise during entirely doctor-centered interviewing.]*

It is this detailed, personal description of symptoms that the interviewer wants at the outset of step 4; it seldom requires more than a few minutes. The interviewer should now understand much of the chronology of symptoms and their descriptive terms (throbbing headache and nausea) that will be expanded upon with the later doctor-centered process, and also the unique personal context in which symptoms occurred, in the patient's own words. By avoiding a focus on the symptoms that inserts information not introduced by the patient ("Did you ever have a head injury?" or "How does the headache affect your vision?") or other diagnostic data with closed-ended questions, the interviewer learns who else was involved, what the patient thought, and generally what was going on in the patient's life. We already have an explanation for her headaches and know what is most bothersome to Mrs. Jones.

While the beginning interviewer may not be aware of this, the physical symptom data given by Mrs. Jones are quite suggestive of migraine headaches; that is, they are throbbing, periodic, and associated with nausea. It is not infrequent that highly diagnostic data for the patient's underlying disease arise during the detailed personal description of symptoms [11]. Indeed, it is the great diagnostic yield here that reportedly led Sir William Osler to say, "Listen to the patient, he is telling you the diagnosis" [12]. Even when symptom data are not diagnostic, the student obtains an overview of the problem, one that does not need to be repeated when switching to the doctor-centered process.

If there are only psychological complaints (no physical symptoms presented), the psychological symptoms are treated in the same way; for example, if Mrs. Jones were complaining of anxiety or feeling blue instead of headaches, the interviewer would determine the personal context of these symptoms, using open-ended queries.

The interviewer thus hears the patient's own description of the symptom data. These data will be expanded to their personal context next, deferring details of symptom data until the interviewer switches to the doctor-centered process in 5 to 10 minutes. It is at the beginning of step 4, however, that the initial integration of symptoms and personal factors must be established in the interviewer's mind, the first view of the patient's mind-body connection. This integration is the core of the interview and the patient-centered process. Most subsequent information in the HPI will be linked to this core. In the next segment, we see how the more general personal aspects of the patient's illness emerge.

Extend the Personal Story to the Broader Context of the Symptoms

The interviewer next learns about the patient and her illness in its broader personal context. This material relates less to symptoms and may be of less diagnostic value for disease but is important to understand illness. In general, the longer the interview, the less the personal data relate to symptoms, and the more they reflect the patient's general life situation. Nonetheless, important diagnostic data can still arise; for example, clues to occupational or drug and alcohol problems. These data will directly influence treatment and prevention programs. One continues to rely upon *focusing open-*

ended skills, focusing them on the patient's personal statements that seem most important to understanding their story.

Direct Continuation of Vignette of Mrs. Jones

PT: I'm on the road a lot. No trouble then either. Except one time when he called me.

DOC: Tell me more about your boss. *[The interviewer encourages discussion of an important personal issue; the student also could have focused on the job itself and accomplished the same goal of obtaining more personal data. Rather than an open-ended request, the interviewer also could have focused the patient by echoing ("he called you") or summarizing the personal aspects; i.e., any of the focusing open-ended skills could be used. They all lead to the same theme.]*

PT: Well, he's been there a long time and I've replaced him in every way there is, except he is still in charge, at least in his title. He yells at everybody. Nobody likes him and he doesn't do much. That's why they got me in there, the Board, so something would get done. These headaches have all come since I got this job — right here. They throb behind my eye and . . . *[Note the corroboration of earlier data: The job is linked to the headaches but Mrs. Jones is now giving additional personal information about her situation that helps the interviewer better understand this connection.]*

DOC: Wait a second, you're getting ahead of me. You say he's in charge but you are the lead attorney? *[Student interrupts respectfully, and then summarizes personal issues to refocus on the job because the patient is going back to physical symptoms already discussed; also the student plans to address symptom details about 5 to 10 minutes from this point, during the doctor-centered process.]*

PT: Yeah, they are phasing him out but he's still there in the meantime. Who knows how long it'll take. I hope I last. *[She is further expanding the story to personal issues less directly related to symptoms, allowing the student to begin to appreciate the nuances and depth of how her job and headaches interact.]*

DOC: Hope you last? *[Echoing will maintain the focus in this area. Note how focusing open-ended skills are used repeatedly to focus the patient, and that they can be applied to the patient's immediately preceding utterances, or they can interrupt them to focus*

*on others previously mentioned—but new data are never intro-
duced to the conversation.]*

In general, a personal focus is easily established as the student
moves away from the immediate personal context of symptoms to
the broader personal context of the patient's illness. A sense of the
patient's personal situation has begun to develop.

Continue to Develop a Free Flow of Personal Data
To maintain the personal focus, the interviewer avoids focusing
back on previously discussed physical complaints. We want to
expand our understanding of the patient as a person. The interviewer relies most on focusing open-ended questions.

Patients occasionally will give their story without much facilita-
tion. Usually, however, they give small bits of personal information, one at a time, as though testing the water to see if the student
is interested, comfortable, and willing to follow them into what is
often new, incompletely recognized material. Because of this step-
by-step unfolding of the story, the interviewer usually must use
focusing open-ended skills repeatedly to draw out the underlying
narrative thread.

Early on, the interviewer focuses on and facilitates whatever bits
of personal data appear to be of most interest to both patient and
student. Once the narrative thread of meaning is identified, the
interviewer stays with this line of inquiry. If the patient gets away
from the central theme, the interviewer interrupts with focusing
open-ended skills and refocuses on the main story thread. Such
refocusing often is necessary because patients tend to wander back
to previously discussed physical symptoms (or other diagnostic or
therapeutic data), perhaps because of unconscious resistance to
personal material or because of the medical setting.

After no more than a few minutes, the interviewer usually has a
good sense of the broader personal story, and has further enhanced the doctor-patient relationship by addressing features of
central importance to the patient's life. If emotions occur during
these early stages, the interviewer often addresses them.

Continuation of Vignette of Mrs. Jones
DOC: Hope you last?
PT: I'm not sure how much of this I can take. They said there
wouldn't be any problem with him and that he would be helpful.
Actually, I kind of liked him at first but then all . . .

DOC: They said? Who are they? *[Interrupts to focus on a bit of information mentioned just before and redirects her to that with echoing; if the interviewer wanted her to simply proceed, an open-ended request would have sufficed, such as "Go on."]*

PT: The Board, they run the company. It's not real big but it's a good chance for someone young like me to get experience in corporate stuff. *[A new layer of data that is not directly related to her headache but provides a deeper understanding of its context]*

DOC: Sounds like the Board told you one thing, that you liked him at first, but then he changed, and you're left with a problem? *[Summarizes what is becoming a free flow of personal data. This is abbreviated for space reasons, but the interviewer ordinarily would further develop this with more focusing open-ended inquiry.]*

Develop an Emotional Focus

Just as the interviewer sought to understand the personal context of the symptoms, he now seeks the emotional context of the personal information. This further deepens the story and makes apparent a three-way interaction among physical, personal, and emotional dimensions. In developing an emotional focus, the interviewer monitors the patient's readiness to engage in this sometimes more stressful discussion by observing how well they are responding to the process and looks for any untoward responses to inquiry about emotion (e.g., changing the subject after the interviewer inquires about emotion).

To establish an emotional focus, the student must *change the style of inquiry. Emotion-seeking skills, both direct and indirect, temporarily replace focusing open-ended skills.* Starting with direct inquiry about how the patient feels concerning the personal situation so far described ("How'd that make you feel?"), the interviewer fully explores the emotional domain. Indirect inquiry using self-disclosure and inquiry about beliefs and impact also may be necessary and is used when direct inquiry does not reveal emotional content. The interviewer should actively elicit emotions. Sometimes the interviewer must make several efforts before emotion can be expressed. As noted, one avoids making the patient uncomfortable.

Emotion-seeking skills are not used when the patient already is showing or expressing emotions, as some will following open-ended inquiry alone.

Continuation of Vignette of Mrs. Jones

DOC: Sounds like the Board told you one thing, that you liked him at first, but then he changed, and you're left with a problem?

PT: Yeah, sounds kind of bad, huh?

DOC: How do you feel about that? *[Direct emotion-seeking]*

PT: Oh, I don't know. The headache is what bothers me.

DOC: But how'd you feel, you know personally, your emotions? *[She didn't give any emotion the first time and interviewer uses direct emotion-seeking inquiry again. It can be appropriate to "push" like this, always monitoring the patient's response and readiness to engage at an emotional level.]*

PT: Oh, nothing really bothers me that much. We were taught to turn the other cheek.

DOC: You know, an old boss of mine once put me in a bind like this. It took me quite awhile but I finally realized I was very upset. *[Interviewer changes strategy and pushes further using self-disclosure, which, of course, must be accurate and genuine.]*

PT: Well, yeah, I guess I am too, now that you mention it.

DOC: What is the feeling? *[She has acknowledged emotion but the interviewer pushes further to get the full picture, returning to a direct emotion-seeking question about feeling.]*

PT: Well, I just want to throw something at him. He makes me so mad. I didn't do anything against him. I work really hard there and things are going much better since I've been there. It's when I get mad that the headaches come. The nausea is even worse and then sometimes I get these spots in my eyes and . . . *[A more precise direct link to headaches, now not just to her job situation but more specifically to being angry. Note the value of pushing for emotion: She is now expressing it.]*

DOC: So you get mad when he gets on you? *[Interspersing open-ended skills is appropriate as the interviewer summarizes to continue this focus.]*

Address the Emotion

When emotions have been expressed, either spontaneously during open-ended inquiry or via the interviewer's use of emotion-seeking skills, yet *another set of skills becomes more important temporarily: the emotion-handling skills outlined in Chapter 2, consisting of Naming, Understanding, Respecting, and Supporting (NURS).*

When emotion is expressed, the interviewer conveys (1) that he has recognized it by naming it, (2) that he understands it, (3) that he respects the patient's plight (or joy), and (4) that he is available to help in any way possible. These skills often are needed several times during the course of an interview. It may take the patient considerable time to work through strong emotional reactions. Using these skills once is seldom enough.

The interviewer occasionally uses emotion-handling skills together as a set, in the order given. Usually, however, only one or two skills are used at a time. Because their excessive use will strike the patient as peculiar or manipulative, one uses them selectively and fits them smoothly and unobtrusively into the conversation.

Emotion-handling skills are used when one has heard enough to adequately understand the emotion. For example, when someone expresses sadness over loss of a spouse, it is not possible to immediately say one understands and appreciates how difficult the situation is. The interviewer must first listen to enough of the story open-endedly to be able to legitimately make these emotion-handling statements. On the other hand, with reticent patients the interviewer may have to use emotion-handling skills with much less emotional information than is desirable. For instance, in a reticent patient who has lost a job and will only acknowledge being "slightly upset," one still uses the NURS quartet actively.

Many interviewers resist emotion-seeking and emotion-handling skills. Some students remark that these skills seem forced and false at first. For those who respond this way, I recommend only that they try. It will indeed feel awkward and phony for many at first but, as self-consciousness is overcome and benefit to the patient observed, most interviewers become rapid converts, recognizing that they feel progressively more comfortable and that their responses are genuine. Many interviewers have had to overcome these same reservations. Because emotions are a basic means of human expression, deep contact with the patient is possible when emotion-seeking and emotion-handling skills are used effectively.

Continuation of Vignette of Mrs. Jones

DOC: So you get mad when he gets on you?

PT: Yeah, he really gets me mad. I just get so furious I could scream sometimes (clenches fist and strikes table firmly).

DOC: It sure makes sense. It seems like you've done so much there to help and all you get is grief from him. I appreciate the way you're able to talk about it. He sure gets you mad. *[The interviewer* *expresses understanding briefly and expresses respect for her by acknowledging she has been through a lot and is successful at work, and by praising her for talking about her emotions. Finally, the interviewer again names the emotion, continuing to use Mrs. Jones' term "mad" rather than "anger" or another more loaded term.]*

PT: He sure does. Just talking about it gets me upset and gives me a headache, right now. *[This further demonstrates the association between headaches and emotional upset, now occurring as a result of anger-laden material in the interview.]*

DOC: I can imagine. You've put up with a lot. *[Naming "mad" again is unnecessary because it's obvious, but the interviewer again indicates understanding and makes a respecting statement.]*

PT: You know, I think I'm even madder at that damn Board. They didn't tell me any of this and said everything would be okay. Who needs all this? *[As a result of addressing her emotions, the patient is now presenting new personal data and its associated emotional material; i.e., the story deepens.]*

DOC: That's a tough situation. *[Interviewer again respects.]*

Use the "Core Dynamic Skills" to Better Identify and Deepen the Story

The student should review the sequence of skills outlined so far in step 4: focusing open-ended skills followed by emotion-seeking skills followed by emotion-handling skills. This typically produces a beginning but still incomplete story. To develop the story further requires the *repetitive, cyclic use of this sequence of skills,* what I call the *core dynamic skills* of the interview. Each cycle produces a deeper level of the story. Personal data and its associated emotion evolve in tandem with neither more important than the other. This deepening of the narrative thread occurs because emotion-handling skills have a powerful facilitative effect on the patient's subsequent expression of new nonemotional, personal information. The interviewer then returns to open-ended inquiry to develop the newly evolving, deeper thread of the story and, later, returns again to emotion-seeking and emotion-handling skills to develop the emotional dimension of the new data. And so on until the interviewer is satisfied with the depth of the story. This self-reinforcing effect of the patient's psychological statements and emotions is key to obtaining the full psychological and emotional story. The interviewer does not focus on just the psychological or just the emotional aspect. One is the context of the other and both are developed nearly simultaneously in a progressive unfolding of the narrative theme.

The story develops spontaneously as the interviewer repeatedly cycles among focusing open-ended, emotion-seeking, and emotion-handling skills. As the patient becomes comfortable in expressing emotion, fewer of the emotion-seeking skills are needed, and emotion-handling and focusing open-ended skills alternate, taking the patient quickly to progressively deeper levels of his story.

In developing the story, the interviewer always will have ideas (hypotheses) about what the story implies. Paradoxically, and distinct from the doctor-centered process, the interviewer does not ask directly about an hypothesis until it has first been mentioned by the patient. For example, if the interviewer thought a patient's story about disliking a woman who "looks like my wife" meant that the patient disliked his wife, the student can't ask directly ("Don't you like your wife?") because it would insert new data (dislike of wife) into the conversation. Rather, the student must get the patient to himself inform this question (e.g., "Tell me more about your wife"). The hypothesis-testing process is analogous to dancing. While the patient leads the dance, once the patient has led to a specific place, the interviewer can maintain a focus on that spot. The interviewer should focus, first open-endedly and then emotionally, on the area where the answer to the hypothesis lies to test a specific hypothesis.

Continuation of Vignette of Mrs. Jones
DOC: . . . That's a tough situation.
PT: You know the head of the Board even told me my boss is a good guy who was looking forward to me coming so he could retire!
DOC: The head of the Board? *[Interviewer now shifts away from emotion-handling to focusing open-ended inquiry with echoing to get what appears to be new information about the situation. This will start a new cycle of active open-ended, emotion-seeking, and emotion-handling skills—the "core dynamic skills."]*
PT: She's the one who recruited me here. I could have gone a couple other places but came here because she convinced me it was such a good chance for me.

DOC: Sounds like you didn't get a full picture of this place? *[Focusing open-ended summary, still trying to learn more new information]*

PT: Yeah, it's not really fair.

DOC: How's that make you feel? *[Now back to emotion with a direct emotion-seeking inquiry]*

PT: Well I must sound kind of stupid, and I feel kind of sheepish. But mostly just mad.

DOC: It makes sense to me, but I don't understand why you feel sheepish. You did everything that you could. *[Back to emotion-handling skills with an understanding statement and respect statement. Notice how open-ended and relationship-building skills are interwoven to generate both nonemotional data and emotions. Notice also that one can indicate lack of understanding and ask for clarification.]*

PT: Yeah, I guess, but I still feel kind of dumb.

DOC: Dumb? *[Echoing. An obvious story is already present but the interviewer is exploring further by again moving away from emotion.]*

PT: That's what my mother used to say, that I was smart but dumb. You know what I mean?

DOC: Smart with books but not so much with people? *[A combination of a summary and an educated guess]*

PT: Yeah, maybe she's right.

DOC: How'd that feel, when she'd say that? *[Back to emotion with direct emotion-seeking]*

PT: Mad! Seems like a pattern, huh? And I used to get headaches as a kid too when she'd get on me. I'd forgotten that. *[Additional supportive data about the association of headaches and anger]*

DOC: So that made you mad too. I'm impressed at how you're able to talk about it and put this together. *[Interviewer uses a naming and a respecting statement. Depending on the time available, the interviewer could have further addressed another obvious clue, the patient's mother, perhaps with an open-ended request such as "Tell me more about your mother." Note in this vignette that another cycle of focusing open-ended, emotion-seeking, and emotion-handling skills has been used to further develop the story. As the interviewer's appreciation of mental mechanisms grows, he will realize that Mrs. Jones is opening up considerably and beginning to reveal basic material about her own growth and development*

process; e.g., her relationship with her mother. With an under-
standing of, for example, Oedipal mechanisms, the inter-
viewer could open-endedly develop deeper understanding of
Mrs. Jones' relationships with her parents and siblings. This,
in turn, helps understand the basic issues in her current life
and, indeed, the relationship between Mrs. Jones and the inter-
viewer. This exciting area of understanding human dy-
namics awaits the student who wants to truly comprehend
human beings.]

Conclude and Address Other Current Issues

If an urgent personal problem exists, easily determined in 5 to 15 minutes, the patient may require additional time, even immediate action. In the absence of an urgent problem, the usual situation, the interviewer begins to conclude the interview when he has an understanding, not of the entire story, but of the most salient, immediate aspects of the patient's story; that is, the first few "chapters". Certainly, there is more to Mrs. Jones' story but, given time constraints and lack of urgency, these areas can be explored another time. The interviewer has a good understanding and, most important, the patient feels understood.

We still have to explore the personal dimension of Mrs. Jones' colitis and recent cough before concluding the initial patient-centered process. The student obtains a personal description of these symptoms and addresses their broader personal context, just as he did with the headaches. Because these are less pressing and troubling, however, usually no more than a few minutes is needed. Nevertheless, although the most problematic issues should have been identified, the student sometimes finds that time-consuming issues arise at this later point and they must, of course, be fully addressed. Careful agenda-setting, however, helps to avoid this.

Continuation of Vignette of Mrs. Jones

DOC: So that made you mad too. I'm impressed at how you're able to talk about it and put this together.

PT: Well, I appreciate your saying that. Actually, it feels kind of good talking. *[A positive response to this interaction]*

DOC: Say more about that. *[An open-ended request]*

PT: Well, I just haven't talked much about it. My husband doesn't want to talk about it.

DOC: He doesn't want to talk? *[Echoing]*

PT: No. I think he feels bad because he thought this was the best place for me to come.

DOC: I'm glad it's been helpful here. You've really been open. *[A support statement followed by a respect statement. An obvious new area for further discussion has been introduced, the patient's husband, and this could be pursued further if time allowed]*

PT: Thanks. My headache's better now. Talking does help.

DOC: I wanted to focus now on your colitis. *[Changes focus]*

PT: Well, it's fine now. I've almost forgotten it.

DOC: What were the symptoms? *[This will allow a personal description of the symptoms]*

PT: Just a little diarrhea everyday. It started when I was under a lot of stress on my job.

DOC: Stress? [Echoing]

PT: Yeah, every time I'd have to go to court I'd have loose stools for a few days before and after. But, I was in court a lot so they were there most of the time. Then the blood began — that scared me — and the hospital. I was okay after that except for a couple minor spells. *[A good overview of the problem and its relationship to the stress of her job, again showing the value of a personal description of symptoms. She views herself as having no problems now and this certainly is not pressing.]*

DOC: That sounds scary but you got some good help. *[Names and identifies prior support.]*

PT: Everyone said they were the best.

DOC: Earlier, you mentioned your parents' reactions to the colitis. *[Open-endedly focusing the patient on material that arose during agenda-setting. Because Mrs. Jones has already mentioned her mother, the interviewer reintroduces this topic to see if it provides additional understanding of the problem; i.e., the student had some inkling (hypothesis) that Mrs. Jones' early history might relate to her present problems.]*

PT: Yeah, they were more upset than I was, especially my mother. I'd never seen her like that.

DOC: Like that? *[Echoing]*

PT: She was so concerned.

DOC: Say more about that. *[Open-ended request]*

PT: She came to see me and did things for me when I was in the hospital. I was okay but you'd never have known it looking at her. She was a wreck.

DOC: How did you feel about that? *[Direct emotion-seeking]*
PT: Kind of good actually. I felt like she cared. She even said she loved me then. That was the first time but she has kept it up some since. We're actually getting along much better since the colitis.
DOC: You smile when you recall that. Sounds like a happy feeling for you. It's nice for you to have support from her. *[Naming and supporting statements. Support does not always have to be from the interviewer; the interviewer can note it from others as well.]*
PT: She's no problem now, it's my boss!
DOC: And the cough? *[Changes focus]*
PT: Well, actually, it's gone now. I was just wondering about it.
DOC: Oh, well we can check that out more later. *[The interviewer would further explore the cough now only if he had had difficulty obtaining personal data earlier and was still trying to get a personal understanding of the patient. The cough can be further analyzed in the doctor-centered HPI or PMH.]*
PT: Yeah, it's really not a problem. We all had it.

Transition to Doctor-Centered Process (Step 5)

Realizing that he will soon enter a more doctor-controlled process, the interviewer anticipates the ending by a minute or so to ensure ending on a positive, supportive note [1]. One can weave the emotion-handling skills into the summary and check the accuracy of the summary. Even in the most desperate situations, the interviewer usually can find something positive and supportive about the patient's situation and provide some hope, even if only one's personal support and availability.

Step 5 is summarized in Table 3-5. The interviewer warns the patient that the content of the interview and, more important, the patient-centered style are about to change. Otherwise, the patient might be confused or taken aback by the doctor-centered style to follow.

Continuation of Vignette with Mrs. Jones
PT: Yeah, it's really not a problem. We all had it.
DOC: So, you're in a new job that hasn't worked out quite like

Table 3-5. Transition to the doctor-centered process (step 5)

1. Brief summary
2. Check accuracy
3. Indicate that both content and style of inquiry will change if the patient is ready

Adapted from Smith RC, Hoppe RB. The patient's story: integrating the patient- and physician-centered approaches to interviewing. *Ann Intern Med* 115:470–477, 1991.

you were led to believe and that has caused you some upset with at least a couple people and quite bad headaches. Do you want to add anything? *[A nice summary. A positive tone to the interaction already exists and nothing further is needed; if the patient were distraught or upset, the interviewer would highlight his and others' support.]*

PT: No, I think you've pretty much got it.

DOC: If it's okay then, I'd like to shift gears and ask you some different types of questions about your headaches and colitis. I'll be asking a lot more questions about specifics. *[The interviewer checks if it is satisfactory to change the subject and indicates what is going to occur.]*

PT: Sure, that's what I came in for.

(Mrs. Jones' story continues in Chapter 5)

Beyond Basic Interviewing

We have begun to develop a clear understanding of the patient as a complex, unique person. Focusing open-ended skills, emotion-seeking skills, and emotion-handling skills are essential vehicles for eliciting the required data, but they are just a few among many tools in the experienced interviewer's armamentarium. In time, the interviewer will need to acquire skills with active, attentive listening if they want to fully "hear" and understand what the patient says [13,14]. Mack Lipkin, Jr. reminds us that prejudices, time pressures, and preoccupation with other issues, for example, can interfere with hearing the patient's story but that interviewers can offset these influences: they prepare for the interview by clearing themselves, much as an athlete or musician might prepare for a performance [14]. The interviewer takes care of pressing personal or professional issues beforehand, relaxes and clears other issues from his mind, and focuses on the patient. This is especially important if one is to listen at multiple levels [13,14], a skill the interviewer can acquire over time as the basics described in this text become more reflexive. Attention to multiple levels means going beyond the obvious content and emotion presented by the patient to consider (1) how they say something, (2) what is left unsaid, and (3) what is implied. This requires attention to subtleties of grammar, syntax, verb tense, changes of subject, nonverbal cues, incongruity in verbal and emotional content, and the understanding of metaphors [14,15]. Changes in these areas are addressed using the same basic skills; for example, "Are you saying you want this now or you wanted it last week"; "I'm confused, I thought we were talking about your husband and now you're talking about your father"; "What do you mean when you keep saying 'my daughter's father'"; "I've noticed you often say, 'You can't win for losing'"; "You talk about how serious this is but you laugh when you say it."

To understand much patient data requires still additional knowledge and skills. As the interviewer's basic skills become reflexive and they become able to attentively listen at multiple levels, an appreciation of psychological defense mechanisms [16] and other unconscious mental mechanisms [17–19], such as slips of the tongue and spontaneous denial [20], becomes essential to better understanding the patient. Beyond this knowledge and skill base, which the student can acquire during psychiatry rotations, an intimate appreciation of different cultures, their values, and their varying means of expression also must occur to more fully understand patients [21–23]; for example, what is the patient's health belief model [21]? These domains are outside the scope of an introductory interviewing text and are considered now only to emphasize that this text is just the beginning. One must supplement basic interviewing skills to better appreciate how humans think, feel, and behave in a complex environment.

Summary

The five steps of the patient-centered process of Integrated Patient-Doctor Interviewing are as follows: setting the stage (step 1), identifying the chief complaint and agenda (step 2), nonfocused interviewing (step 3), focused interviewing (step 4), and the transition (step 5). In conducting the more difficult steps 3 and 4, the interviewer orchestrates [14] the patient's personal story using the following tools: nonfocusing and focusing open-ended inquiry, occasional closed-ended questions, emotion-seeking and emotion-handling skills, and hypothesis-testing. The cyclic use of the core dynamic skills produces successful patient-centered interviewing and occupies all of the longest and most important step 4. These are the tools that will allow the interviewer to understand the depths of the human condition.

The most difficult part of the interview has been conducted; the data generated are easily understood and usually explain the personal context of physical symptoms. The mind-body connection is established, data that will lead to an integrated biopyschosocial story have begun to emerge, and the patient feels understood.

References

1. Smith RC, Hoppe RB. The patient's story: integrating the patient- and physician-centered approaches to interviewing. *Ann Intern Med* 115: 470–477, 1991.
2. Morgan WL, Engel GL. *The Clinical Approach to the Patient*. Philadelphia: Saunders, 1969.
3. Lipkin JM, et al. Performing the Interview. In Lipkin M, Putnam M, Lazare A (eds.), *The Medical Interview*. New York: Springer-Verlag, 1995. Pp. 65–82.
4. White J, Levinson W, Roter D. "Oh, by the Way . . .": The closing moments of the medical visit. *J Gen Intern Med* 9:24–28, 1994.
5. Barrows HS, Pickell GC. *Developing Clinical Problem-Solving Skills—A Guide to More Effective Diagnosis and Treatment*. New York: Norton Medical Books, 1991.
6. Kravitz RL, et al. Internal medicine patients' expectations for care during office visits. *J Gen Intern Med* 9:75–81, 1994.
7. Platt FW. *Conversation Failure: Case Studies in Doctor-Patient Communication*. Tacoma, WA: Life Sciences Press, 1992.
8. Beckman HB, Frankel RM. The effect of physician behavior on the collection of data. *Ann Intern Med* 101:692–696, 1984.
9. Carson CA. *A Course in Nonverbal Communication for Medical Education*. Rochester, NY: Cecile A. Carson, The Genesee Hospital, Rochester, NY, 1988.
10. Levinson D. *A Guide to the Clinical Interview*. Philadelphia: Saunders, 1987.
11. Cox A, Rutter M, Holbrook D. Psychiatric interviewing techniques V. Experimental study: eliciting factual information. *Br J Psychiatry* 139:29–37, 1981.

12. Jackson SW. The listening healer in the history of psychological healing. *Am J Psychiatry* 149:1623–1632, 1992.
13. Reik T. *Listening With The Third Ear: The Inner Experience of a Psychoanalyst*. New York: Farrar, Straus and Giroux, 1948.
14. Lipkin M. The Medical Interview and Related Skills. In Branch WT (ed.), *Office Practice of Medicine*. Philadelphia: Saunders, 1987. Pp. 1287–1306.
15. Feldman SS. *Mannerisms of Speech and Gestures in Everyday Life*. New York: International Universities Press, 1959.
16. Vaillant GE. Theoretical hierarchy of adaptive ego mechanisms: A 30 year follow-up of 30 men selected for psychological health. *Arch Gen Psychiatry* 24:107–118, 1971.
17. Fenichel O. *The Psychoanalytical Theory of Neurosis*. New York: WW Norton, 1945.
18. Brenner C. *An Elementary Textbook of Psychoanalysis* (revised ed). Garden City, NY: Anchor Press/Doubleday, 1964.
19. Fancher RE. *Psychoanalytic Psychology: The Development of Freud's Thought*. New York: WW Norton, 1973.
20. Freud S. *A General Introduction to Psychoanalysis* (authorized English translation of the revised ed.). New York: Washington Square Press, 1952.
21. Kleinman A, Eisenberg L, Good B. Culture, illness and care—Clinical lessons from anthropologic and cross-culture research. *Ann Intern Med* 88:251–258, 1978.
22. Jenkins JH, Karno M. The meaning of expressed emotion: Theoretical issues raised by cross-cultural research. *Am J Psychiatry* 149:9–21, 1992.
23. Johnson TM, Hardt EJ, Kleinman A. Cultural Factors in the Medical Interview. In Lipkin M, Putnam SM, Lazare A (eds.), *The Medical Interview*. New York: Springer-Verlag, 1995. Pp. 153–162.

Symptom-Defining Skills

With the patient-centered process of Integrated Patient-Doctor Interviewing behind us, we now begin a major transition to the doctor-centered process. Before discussing its specific conduct, however, the new skills it requires must be addressed. These are considered individually in this chapter and synthesized in Chapter 5 as the doctor-centered process.

During the doctor-centered process, multiple bits of information are processed by the physician and briefly addressed with open-ended requests (focused on a specific topic); diagnostic details are then pinned down with many closed-ended questions. This coning-down process occurs repeatedly until all the multiple areas within the HPI/OCAP, HI, PMH, FH, SH, and ROS have been covered. Many of the required details the interviewer must elicit concern symptoms. The interviewer focuses the coning-down process in two categories: (1) developing a common language of symptoms, and (2) further refining these symptoms into more precise data. The symptom-defining skills presented in this chapter describe this process.

Developing a Common Language for All Symptoms

Translating Complaints into Specific Medical Symptoms Is Sometimes Necessary

Patients often speak in nonmedical terms that must be converted to medically meaningful terms. The following is an example of common complaints that need conversion to medically meaningful symptoms. When the interviewer hears that the patient has the "blahs," a "wrung-out feeling," or "bad blood," what does that

---

Common Complaints Needing Conversion
to Symptoms in the System Review

Blahs
Dragged-out
Bad blood
I've got a "bunch"
Really weird
Funny smelling urine
Wrung-out
Midlife crisis
Menopause
Old age
Terrible 2s
A rod in my head
Wigged-out
Sun troubles
Chronic fatigue syndrome
Heart murmur
Indigestion
The flu
Dizzy
Allergies

---

mean? and how is the information to be used medically? As shown in the example, a brief open-ended question (focused on the symptom) is followed by enough closed-ended questions to adequately understand the patient's meaning.

> **DOC:** Say more about what you mean by the blahs. *[A focused, open-ended request]*
>
> **PT:** Well, you know, the nausea all the time and no appetite. *[Nausea and no appetite are medically meaningful terms—medical symptoms]*
>
> **DOC:** Any vomiting? *[Closed-ended question]*
>
> **PT:** No.
>
> **DOC:** How's your weight been? *[The interviewer would continue to pursue this to better define what the patient calls the "blahs" but has already identified at least two medical symptoms.]*

Likewise, many medical terms are ambiguous or are used by patients in widely varying, often unconventional ways. To give just one example, "dizzy" usually means vertigo, a sensation of whirling, as though one had just gotten off a merry-go-round or had too much to drink. But, some physicians and many laypersons use the term *dizziness* to mean a faint or light-headed feeling unattended by vertigo. This distinction is important because one approaches the patient with vertigo differently from the patient who is light-headed.

> **DOC:**   Tell me what you mean by dizzy. *[Focused, open-ended request; this could also be phrased as a question like, "What do you mean by dizzy?"]*
>
> **PT:**   I get wobbly on my feet. *[Still not very specific]*
>
> **DOC:**   Do you get a sensation of whirling about, like you'd just stepped off a merry-go-round? *[Closed-ended question to get necessary details]*
>
> **PT:**   Yeah, that's it. I feel like I'm going around the room.
>
> **DOC:**   Do you feel lightheaded, like you might faint or have to put your head down between your knees to get relief? *[Closed-ended inquiry for more details]*
>
> **PT:**   No, that makes it worse to put my head down. *[The interviewer has identified the medical symptom vertigo as the meaning of the complaint of dizziness, although many more questions remain about associated symptoms and other details of the problem. One must always understand what the patient means for a particular symptom.]*

The System Review (Review of Systems [ROS]) Lists the Symptoms of Most Diseases

The system review, the original purpose of which is explained in Chapter 5, is significant here because it lists and organizes the symptoms for most diseases. Symptoms are important because they are the common language through which, in large part, the interviewer converts a patient's complaints to a disease diagnosis. The following outline lists isolated symptoms according to the body system they are associated with, although many occur in more than one system. Neither the common complaints given on p. 56 nor the system review outline are exhaustive. Preclinical students should not worry if they don't understand what symptoms signify about underlying diseases. Symptoms are not diagnostic of the possible disease explanations given in italics, which simply are examples of associations that occur. Diseases can be identified only after enough data have been obtained and synthesized by the

System Review (ROS) With Examples of Some Symptoms*
1. General
    a. Poor appetite [cancer, hepatitis, AIDS, medications, depression]
    b. Excessive appetite [uncontrolled diabetes, hyperthyroidism, depression]
    c. Weight loss [AIDS, cancer, emphysema, chronic infection, depression]
    d. Weight gain [overeating, hypothyroidism, fluid retention]
    e. Fever, chills, sweats [infection]
    f. No enjoyment of life (anhedonia) [depression]
    g. Pain [many causes]
    h. Fatigue, lack of energy [many causes]
2. Integument-related
    a. Sores [infection, trauma, vascular insufficiency, diabetes, self-induced]
    b. Itching (pruritis) [bites, allergy, medications, dry skin, anxiety]
    c. Rash [medications, measles, German measles, chicken pox]
    d. Change in size or color of moles [malignant melanoma]
    e. Abnormal hair growth [adrenal tumor, steroid medications]
    f. Changes in nails [infection, iron deficiency, hypoxia, nail-biting]
3. Hematopoietic
    a. Enlarged glands (lymphadenopathy) [infection, leukemia, infectious mononucleosis, lymphoma]
    b. Lumps anywhere [lipoma, trauma, metastatic or primary cancer]
    c. Urge to eat dirt (pica) or ice [iron deficiency, psychosis]
    d. Abnormal bleeding or excessive bruising [liver disease, leukemia, idiopathic thrombocytopenic purpura, medications]
    e. Frequent or unusual infections [AIDS, diabetes, immunological deficiency, self-induced]
4. Endocrine
    a. Heat intolerance [hyperthyroidism, excessive thyroid medication]
    b. Cold intolerance [hypothyroidism, weight loss]
    c. Decreased sexual drive (libido) [hypogonadism, medications, depression]
    d. Salt craving [adrenocortical insufficiency, salt loss]
    e. Enlarging glove and hat size [acromegaly]

f. Excessive thirst (polydipsia) *[uncontrolled diabetes, water loss]*

5. Musculoskeletal

   a. Frequent fractures *[osteoporosis, osteogenesis imperfecta, metastatic cancer, trauma]*

   b. Muscular weakness *[polymyositis, old polio or stroke, electrolyte imbalance]*

   c. Painful muscles *[trichinosis, polymyalgia rheumatica, muscle strain]*

   d. Joint pain and swelling *[osteoarthritis, rheumatoid arthritis, gout]*

   e. Low back pain *[psychogenic, herniated disk, muscle strain, infection, tumor]*

   f. Paralysis *[stroke, polio, head injury]*

   g. Movement difficulty *[Parkinson's disease, medications]*

   h. Pain in calf with walking (intermittent claudication) *[vascular insufficiency, muscle strain]*

   i. Swollen leg *[trauma, varicosities, venous stasis, thrombophlebitis, infection, chronic dependent positioning]*

6. Eyes, ears, nose, and throat

   a. Change in vision *[aging, diabetes, glaucoma, foreign body, stroke, brain tumor]*

   b. Spots in visual field *[migraine, glaucoma]*

   c. Double vision (diplopia) *[brain tumor, stroke]*

   d. Loss of hearing *[aging, ear wax, tumor]*

   e. Ringing in the ears (tinnitus) *[Meniere's disease, tumor, aging]*

   f. Drainage from nose *[common cold, cerebrospinal fluid rhinorrhea, allergy]*

   g. Decreased or altered sense of smell *[brain tumor, rhinitis]*

   h. Bloody nose (epistaxis) *[trauma, tumor, infection]*

   i. Sore throat *[bacterial or viral infection, psychogenic, medication-induced]*

   j. Impaired speech *[stroke, tumor, cleft lip or palate, psychogenic]*

   k. Painful tooth *[cavity (caries), abscess, trauma]*

   l. Hoarseness *[laryngeal cancer, voice abuse, polyps]*

7. Head and neck

   a. Headache *[tension, migraine, brain tumor, medications]*

   b. Dizzy (vertigo) *[labyrinthitis, tumor, vertebral-basilar insufficiency, medications]*

    c.   Light-headedness *[psychogenic, anemia, fluid/electrolyte disturbance, rapid standing (orthostatic)]*

    d.   Loss of consciousness (syncope) *[orthostatic, aortic stenosis, rapid bleeding, cardiac arrhythmia, cerebrovascular accident, trauma, stress-related]*

    e.   Stiff neck *[arthritis, muscle strain, cervical disk]*

8. Breasts
   a. Lump or mass *[cancer, fibrocystic disease, abscess, trauma]*
   b. Discharge *[cancer, medications, lactation]*
   c. Tenderness *[menstrual, medications]*

9. Cardiovascular and pulmonary
   a. Chest pain *[pneumonia, muscular strain, coronary artery disease, pulmonary embolus, psychogenic, pericarditis, pleurisy]*
   b. Shortness of breath (dyspnea) *[see most of chest pain (a.); also heart failure, anemia]*
   c. Shortness of breath when lying down and need to sit to breathe (orthopnea) *[heart failure, emphysema, pneumonia]*
   d. Wakening at night with dyspnea (paroxysmal nocturnal dyspnea) *[heart failure, emphysema, sleep apnea]*
   e. Wheezing *[asthma, heart failure, pulmonary embolus, cancer, foreign body, upper airway obstruction]*
   f. Cough *[see most of above]*
   g. Yellow or green sputum *[bronchitis, pneumonia]*
   h. Clear sputum *[heart failure, asthma]*
   i. Bloody sputum (hemoptysis) *[pneumonia, pulmonary embolus, heart failure, cancer]*
   j. Pounding sensation in chest (palpitations) *[arrhythmias, ventricular hypertrophy, tachycardia]*
   k. (See Musculoskeletal and 2. Integument-related for peripheral arterial and venous insufficiency)

10. Gastrointestinal
    a. (See 1. General for appetite and weight changes)
    b. Sticking sensation in throat (globus hystericus) *[stress-related, foreign body, infection]*
    c. Difficulty swallowing (dysphagia) *[achalasia, cancer, esophagitis, foreign body]*
    d. Heartburn *[esophagitis, medications, cancer]*
    e. Upper abdominal pain *[gastritis, peptic ulcer disease, medications, psychogenic, gallbladder disease, pancreatitis, abdominal wall pain]*
    f. Mid-lower abdominal pain *[appendicitis, diverticulitis,*

irritable bowel syndrome, cancer, vascular insufficiency, Meckel's diverticulum, regional enteritis, ulcerative colitis]

g. Nausea *[many of the above; medications, hepatitis]*
h. Nonbloody vomiting (emesis) *[many of the above]*
i. Bloody emesis (hematemesis) *[upper gastrointestinal bleeding: esophagitis, gastritis, ulcer, cancer]*
j. Black stools (melena) *[upper gastrointestinal bleeding]*
k. Bloody stools (hematochezia) *[rapid upper gastrointestinal bleeding or lower gastrointestinal bleeding: hemorrhoids, cancer, vascular insufficiency, diverticulitis, vascular anomalies, ulcerative colitis]*
l. Difficult or infrequent bowel movements (constipation) *[cancer, hypothyroidism, medications, diverticulitis, low-fiber diet]*
m. Loose or frequent bowel movements (diarrhea) *[infection, diverticulitis, cancer, medications, ulcerative colitis, excessive dietary fiber]*
n. Yellow discoloration of sclerae and skin (jaundice) *[hepatitis, biliary obstruction, medications, hemolytic anemias]*
o. Dark urine like tea or a cola drink *[see jaundice (n.) except obstruction]*
p. Excessive upper (belching or eructation) or lower (flatus) bowel gas *[many of the above; swallowing air when eating fast, high-fiber diet]*
q. Rectal pain (proctalgia), discharge, or itching (pruritis ani) *[psychogenic, hygienic, hemorrhoids, fissure, infection (gonorrhea or pinworm)]*
r. Lump in groin or scrotum *[hernia, lymphadenopathy]*

11. Urinary
a. Increased urinary frequency (polyuria) *[infection, bladder neck obstruction, excessive water intake, diabetes]*
b. Burning with urination (dysuria) *[infection]*
c. Getting up more than once during the night to void (nocturia) *[infection, bladder neck obstruction, excessive fluid intake]*
d. Need to urinate suddenly and urgently (urgency) *[infection]*
e. Loss of urinary control (incontinence) *[brain or spinal cord lesion, infection, stress incontinence]*
f. Bloody urine (hematuria) *[infection, cancer, kidney stone, bladder polyps]*

   g. Particulate matter in urine *[stones, small stony debris (gravel), sloughed renal papillae]*
   h. Slow to get urinary stream started (hesitancy) *[bladder neck obstruction]*
12. Genital, male
   a. Urethral discharge *[gonorrhea and other infections]*
   b. Penile sores or growth *[syphilis and other infections, cancer]*
   c. Painful or swollen testicle *[cancer, epididymitis, orchitis, trauma, hernia, hydrocele, spermatocele]*
   d. Impotence *[psychogenic, diabetes, vascular disease, medications]*
   e. Bloody ejaculation (hematospermia) *[prostatitis, tumor]*
   f. Retrograde ejaculation into bladder *[diabetes, autonomic dysfunction]*
   g. Premature ejaculation *[psychogenic, prostatitis]*
   h. Decreased libido *[psychogenic, chronic illness, medications]*
13. Genital, female
   a. Vaginal discharge or itching *[gonorrhea or other infection, foreign body, fistula, irritant-induced]*
   b. Sores or lumps *[syphilis or other infection, cancer, abscess]*
   c. Painful menses (dysmenorrhea) *[pelvic inflammatory disease, endometriosis, cancer]*
   d. Absence of menses (amenorrhea) *[pregnancy, lactation, malnutrition, menopause, medications, endocrine]*
   e. Irregular, heavy menses (menometrorrhagia) *[medications, endocrine, endometriosis, pelvic inflammatory disease]*
   f. Hot flashes *[menopause, ovarian failure]*
   g. Decreased libido *[see 4. Endocrine]*
   h. Painful intercourse (dyspareunia) *[endometriosis, pelvic inflammatory disease]*
   i. Nonorgasmic *[chronic illness, psychogenic]*
14. Neuropsychiatric
   a. (See 6. Eyes, ears, nose, and throat and 7. Head and neck for cranial nerves)
   b. (See 5. Musculoskeletal for motor)
   c. Numb, tingling sensation in extremities (paresthesia) *[neuritis, tumor, disk]*
   d. Decreased (hypesthesia) or absent (anesthesia) sensation *[neuritis, disk, tumor]*
   e. Tremor *[Parkinson's disease, anxiety, tumor, medications]*
   f. Loss of balance *[labyrinthine disease, tumor, stroke, visual, infection]*

g. Difficulty walking (ataxia) [*Parkinson's disease, stroke, tumor, neuritis, head injury*]

h. Seizures [*epilepsy, tumor, stroke, medications, infection, vitamin deficiency*]

i. Bizarre, unrealistic thoughts (intrusive thoughts) [*psychosis, head injury, medications or street drugs, drug-alcohol withdrawal, depression, dementia*]

j. Bizarre, unrealistic perceptions (hallucinations) [*see i. above*]

k. Depression [*psychiatric, chronic disease, medications*]

l. Mania [*manic-depressive, medications, hyperthyroidism*]

m. Poor judgment, orientation, memory, attention, and concentration [*see i. above, psychogenic*]

n. Inability to get to sleep or stay asleep (insomnia) [*depression, psychogenic, sleep apnea, medications, drug-alcohol use and withdrawal, nocturnal myoclonus, chronic disease*]

o. Hypersomnolence [*depression, sleep apnea, narcolepsy, medications, insufficient sleep, tumor, infection, head injury, chronic diseases*]

p. Nighmares [*depression, severe stress, medications*]

q. Anhedonia [*see 1. General*]

r. Suicidal [*depression, other psychiatric, medications, chronic disease*]

s. Anxiety, nervousness [*stress, depression, hyperthyroidism, medications or drugs, panic disorder*]

t. Symptoms without an explanation (somatization) [*normal variant, personality disorder*]

---

*Many of these symptoms can occur in systems other than where listed and, in addition to those listed, there are many other diseases and disorders that can cause these symptoms. Terms listed in parentheses are synonyms.

Adapted from Morgan WL, Engel GL. *The Clinical Approach to the Patient.* Philadelphia: Saunders, 1969, and Billings AJ, Stoeckle JD. *The Clinical Encounter: A Guide to the Medical Interview and Case Presentation.* Chicago: Year Book, 1989.

---

student. Medical terminology for some symptoms also is noted in parentheses. Preclinical students are urged to learn all 14 categories and to know a few symptoms in each. Clinical-level students will learn and develop understanding of all symptoms during clinical rotations. They are urged to memorize all symptoms in each category, a necessary prerequisite for effective doctor-centered interviewing [1]. The interviewer must know and understand the language into which she translates the patient's complaints. It is the basis for diagnosis and treatment.

Distinguishing Closely Related Material from Symptoms

The patient directly experiences symptoms and is therefore the only authority on his own symptoms; no verification is necessary (e.g., abdominal pain and diarrhea). This defines so-called *primary data* [2]. Away from a patient's direct experience, data are less reliable and more in need of verification (e.g., "The doctor said it was appendicitis"). Thus, nonsymptom disease information obtained from the patient (such as a diagnosis, treatment, procedure, medication, cause of the problem, or a laboratory test) differs from the patient's actual symptoms. While these *secondary data* are less important [2], they often guide the interviewer to areas requiring verification and additional information. Incorporation of secondary data into the interview is described in Chapter 5.

Symptoms are distinguished from "signs" in medicine. The patient complains about a symptom (chest pain, dyspnea) while the interviewer or patient observes a sign on physical examination (tender ribs, heart murmur). Symptoms and signs occasionally overlap, as in a patient complaining of "yellow jaundice" and the interviewer observing that the patient is jaundiced. Students learn about signs in physical diagnosis courses and on clinical rotations.

Refining Individual Symptoms into more Precise Data

Once a symptom is identified, the interviewer can make the symptom descriptions more precise to improve their meaningfulness for diagnosing diseases. Greater specificity derives from the set of descriptors outlined here and often requires mostly closed-ended inquiry. As before, examples given in text are not exhaustive and more data are needed to make a final diagnosis.

The following descriptors should be sought to the extent possible for each individual symptom. These descriptors reflect the "classic seven" dimensions of symptoms: body location, quality, quantitation, chronology and timing, setting, moderating factors (aggravating/alleviating), and associated symptoms [3,4]; nonpain symptoms usually do not require all seven descriptors.

The Seven Descriptors of Symptoms
1. Location and radiation
   a. Precise location
   b. Deep/superficial
   c. Specific/diffuse
2. Quality
   a. Usual descriptors
   b. Unusual descriptors
3. Quantitation
   a. Type of onset
   b. Intensity/severity
   c. Impairment/disability
   d. Numerical description
      (1) Number of events
      (2) Size
      (3) Volume
4. Chronology and timing—course of individual symptom over time
   a. Time of onset of symptom and intervals between its occurrence
   b. Duration of symptom
   c. Periodicity and frequency of symptom
   d. Course of symptom
      (1) Short-term
      (2) Long-term
5. Setting
6. Moderating factors
   a. Precipitants/aggravating
   b. Relieving
7. Associated symptoms

Adapted from Morgan WL, Engel GL. *The Clinical Approach to the Patient*. Philadelphia: Saunders, 1969, and Billings AJ, Stoeckle JD. *The Clinical Encounter: A Guide to the Medical Interview and Case Presentation*. Chicago: Year Book Medical Publishers, 1989.

Location of the Symptom and Its Radiation

The precise location of a symptom is given when possible. Both the location and area of radiation of the symptom can have diagnostic significance; for example, left temporal headache without radiation (*nonspecific*), substernal pain radiating into the neck, jaw, and left arm (*angina, esophagitis*), low back pain radiating into the left buttock and posterior thigh with extension into the lateral aspect of the calf and over the dorsum of the foot into the great toe *(L5-S1 nerve root impingement from a herniated lumbar disk)*. If they do not do so automatically, patients should be asked to point to their area of discomfort; for example, numbness on the ulnar portions of the hand suggests irritation in a C8-T1 nerve root distribution.

Does the patient feel the distress deep or on the surface? Is it specific in location or more diffuse?; for example, left temporal headache localized to the region of the temporal artery that was located by the patient as "on the surface" *(temporal arteritis, skin problem)*.

The student begins this inquiry with a focused, open-ended request, which also can be phrased as a question such as, "Can you describe the location for me?" Closed-ended inquiry usually is needed to get sufficient specificity.

> **DOC:** So, as part of the blahs you've got this stomach pain. Can you describe its location for me? *[A focused open-ended request, phrased as a question, to be followed by several closed-ended questions]*
>
> **PT:** It's in my stomach.
>
> **DOC:** Where exactly is it? Point at it, if you can. *[Always be as specific as possible]*
>
> **PT:** (points to upper midabdomen, the epigastrium)
>
> **DOC:** How big an area? Can you draw a circle around it?
>
> **PT:** (draws an outline) This big.
>
> **DOC:** Does it move anywhere else, like your back or chest? *[Giving examples is helpful as long as the answer is not suggested.]*
>
> **PT:** No.
>
> **DOC:** Is it deep down or feel more like it's right on the surface?
>
> **PT:** Down inside.

Quality of the Symptom

Additional diagnostic specificity sometimes derives from knowing what the symptom feels like; for example, aching *(nonspecific)*, burning *(gastritis or ulcer disease when substernal or epigastric)*, sharp *(nonspecific)*, dull *(nonspecific)*, crushing *(coronary insufficiency when substernal)*, throbbing *(migraine when in head, localized infection anywhere)*, or cramping *(disorder of a hollow organ such as the ureter, intestine, or uterus)*.

Unusual descriptions can signify psychological problems or stress, and can sometimes be understood metaphorically [5]. For example, psychotic people have said such things as "it feels like my intestines have grown shut" or "it feels like they left an instrument in there." Similarly, comments like "it's pushing up through my soul and tearing my heart out" are extraordinary and suggest the presence of some associated psychological issues.

One learns the quality of the symptom by starting with a focused, open-ended request such as, "Tell me what the pain is like." More closed-ended inquiry may be necessary to pin down details.

> **DOC:** What does it feel like? *[A focused open-ended request, again phrased as a question]*
> **PT:** Pretty bad.
> **DOC:** Well, how would you describe it: aching, sharp, dull? *[It is appropriate, if necessary, to give examples as long as an answer is not suggested]*
> **PT:** Kind of burning, like hot or on fire.

Quantitation of the Symptom
Further precision and specificity for disease diagnosis can be gained by quantifying the symptom in the following ways.

Type of Onset
Whether the symptom began gradually or suddenly has diagnostic significance; the latter suggests an acute but not necessarily more important disease process. One might hear, for example, "the weakness just gradually developed in my shoulders and thighs over a couple months" *(polymyositis)*; "the shortness of breath had been kind of gradual over that day but the chest pain and coughing blood came all of a sudden" *(pulmonary embolus, heart failure)*.

Focused open-ended inquiry often suffices, although patients sometimes benefit from giving examples; for example, "Would you tell me how this began?"

> **DOC:** How did this begin?
> **PT:** What do you mean?
> **DOC:** You know, slow or all of a sudden?
> **PT:** Gradual, a little bit at a time.

Intensity

The interviewer obtains a measure of intensity or severity by asking for comparisons to prior experiences (toothache, having a baby) or getting a rating on a 1 to 10 scale where a 10 rating is the worst ever. In general, the more severe the symptom, the more serious the problem. Lower grade pain, however, does not signify an unimportant problem; for example, angina pectoris reflects serious disease but the pain is not always severe. In addition, certain pains are characteristically more severe than others; for example, testicular injury, renal calculus, labor pains.

The interviewer begins open-endedly with a question like, "Give me an idea how bad it was." Usually, however, closed-ended questions are necessary to get the needed details.

DOC: Tell me how severe it is.
PT: Well, it wasn't too bad.
DOC: On a 1 to 10 scale, where 10 is the worst ever, how would you rate it?
PT: Not so bad, really. I guess a 3.
DOC: How is it compared to a toothache?
PT: Not that bad.

Impairment or Disability Resulting from the Symptom

Another measure of severity is how the complaint has affected the patient on a daily basis. For example, a minor episode of hoarseness could work severe hardship on an opera singer or public speaker while it would be of little consequence to a writer or night watchman.

The interviewer again begins with a focused, open-ended request such as, "What effect is this having on your life?" Closed-ended questions are used for detail. Specific inquiry about what the patient is no longer able to do helps clarify the situation; for example, "Since the chest pain started, what have you had to give up?" Comparing the patient's daily activities before and after the symptom further clarifies this. Many of these data will often have been obtained during the patient-centered process and, if so, they are not repeated.

DOC: How's this affecting what you do?
PT: Well, it's caused a lot of problems.
DOC: Is it keeping you off work or anything? *[Note the continued need for closed-ended questions to get accurate details]*

PT: No, nothing like that really. I haven't missed a day of work. I'm just getting tired of it.

Obtain Numerical Data Where Possible
The total number of occurrences of the symptom usually can be identified or closely estimated by the interviewer; for example, there have been about twenty such episodes of chest pain in the last week after no more than one weekly during the preceding year. It also can be necessary to precisely quantify symptoms in other ways when applicable; for example, "It swells to the size of a softball at times but then goes back down to like a golfball" *(inguinal hernia)*; "Only passed about a glassful of urine all day" *(bladder neck obstruction, dehydration)*. The interviewer will find that patients seldom respond with precise numbers, preferring "quite a bit" or "not too much" to precise quantities. It is the interviewer's job to elicit more specific information without alienating the patient.

These data are obtained almost entirely by closed-ended inquiry. The interviewer often has to follow up on answers that are not precise enough; for example, upon being asked how many times a pain occurs, the patient answers "a lot" to which the interviewer might respond, "Can you be more specific, you know, how many times in a day?"

DOC: How many times a day do you have the pain?
PT: Oh, three or four or five.
DOC: What's the most you've had?
PT: Seven or eight times.
DOC: And the least?
PT: One or even none sometimes.

Chronology and Timing — Course of Individual Symptom over Time
The interviewer must learn the precise sequence of symptoms and other events to be most effective diagnostically. Here we will focus on the chronology and timing of individual symptoms; these data will be integrated into the overall chronology of all symptoms in Chapter 5.

Time of Onset and Intervals Between Occurrences
The time of onset of the symptom and the time intervals between occurrences of the symptom have considerable diagnostic signifi-

cance; for example, the onset of a cough 6 months earlier that recurs at intervals of 1 to 2 days suggests a chronic pulmonary problem such as cancer or tuberculosis, while the onset of a cough 2 days earlier that is continuous suggests an acute process such as bronchitis or pneumonia. Recalling Mrs. Jones from the last chapter, migraine headaches characteristically have specific times of onset and pain-free intervals of days to weeks, as contrasted to usually daily and nonremitting headaches from a brain tumor or from tension headaches.

Duration
The duration of a symptom also is of diagnostic significance. Precise understanding is essential; for example, a few seconds, 5 minutes, 2 hours, 10 days, 3 years. Typical substernal crushing pain of coronary disease lasting only 5 to 10 minutes suggests angina pectoris without myocardial infarction (heart attack) while a similar pain lasting an hour or so suggests myocardial infarction. Migraine headaches typically last from 1 to 12 hours, again in contrast to the more constant headaches of a brain tumor or tension headaches.

Periodicity and Frequency
Symptoms often have patterns reflecting the underlying disease process that are of diagnostic importance. For example, the symptoms of different types of malaria occur at distinctive and sometimes diagnostic frequencies. Body cycles also can affect symptoms; for example, premenstrual syndrome focuses around menses and nocturnal myoclonus occurs during nonrapid eye movement sleep. In addition, external influences can have a cyclic impact; for example, regular stressful events, disorders such as allergies and acid peptic disease that have a seasonal association.

Course
The course of the symptom over an individual episode and its pattern of occurrence over a longer period are essential diagnostic data. The individual course of pain stemming from obstruction of a hollow organ is that of a progressive increase in pain followed by apparent relief, often described as cramping, only to be followed at varying intervals by recurrence of the same pattern (e.g., labor pains, ureteral colic). A migraine headache, on the other hand, typically pursues a slow but progressive buildup of a constant throbbing pain.

The overall course of a symptom is equally important, as described more extensively in Chapter 5. A patient with headaches of 20 years duration that are unchanged seldom will have a brain tumor while a progressively worsening headache over several months is suggestive of a tumor or other intracerebral disease process.

The following chronological description is obtained almost entirely with closed-ended questions.

DOC: When did the burning in the stomach begin?
PT: About a year ago. *[Onset]*
DOC: Do you have pain every day?
PT: No, sometimes it will be gone for weeks at a time. *[Intervals between symptom]*
DOC: And how long do they last each time?
PT: Quite a while.
DOC: How long is that? I need a little more detail.
PT: Oh, I don't know. Maybe a couple hours.
DOC: What's the shortest they might last and the longest?
PT: Well, some of them are gone in just a few minutes. But most are about an hour I guess.
DOC: What's the longest?
PT: The worst one I ever had lasted from supper until just about bedtime, about 4 hours. *[Longest and shortest duration of symptom]*
DOC: What seems to determine that?
PT: I don't know, but it's always worse in the spring, and it's not there on weekends when I'm not working. *[Frequency and periodicity]*
DOC: What's the course of the pain with each episode?
PT: It just gradually comes on and then gets a little worse. *[Short-term course of symptom]*
DOC: Overall, how is the pain doing?
PT: It seems worse to me.
DOC: How's that?
PT: Well, it's not more pain, but it's more often. It used to be just once every day or so but now it's four or five times a day. *[Overall course of symptom]*

Setting

If not already obtained during the patient-centered process, the setting in which symptoms occur usually is described as part of obtaining patients' chronological descriptions or as part of learning their functional impairment from the symptom. If this does not happen, the interviewer determines it with questions such as, "Where were you?" or "Who else was present?" or "What were you doing?" or "Where was this?".

One begins open-endedly with questions like, "Can you tell me the background of the symptom, you know, what you were doing at the time and who was there?" If this does not suffice, closed-ended inquiry can help.

> **DOC:** Can you give me some of the background for the pain, like who's around and where you are when it happens?
> **PT:** Almost always at work—there's been a lot of stress lately.
> **DOC:** Not at home?
> **PT:** Never. Isn't that funny?
> **DOC:** Who's around at work?
> **PT:** Well, it's just since I transferred to the parts department *[If these data have not been explicated during the patient-centered process, as part of the personal dimension of the illness, they would be further developed here.]*

Moderating Factors

To this point the interviewer has addressed just the symptom per se, but she now considers some external influences of diagnostic value: precipitants of the problem, what aggravates it once present, and what relieves it. For example, aspirin, alcohol, tobacco, spicy foods, and caffeine all are known to both precipitate and aggravate gastritis or acid peptic disease, while relief is typically obtained by drinking milk, eating bland food, and using antacids. Similarly, angina is precipitated and aggravated by exertion, mental stress, or cold air blowing in the face, while it is relieved, usually in less than 10 minutes, by rest and the use of nitroglycerin.

While one begins open-endedly, most of this information occurs through closed-ended questioning, the specific content of which reflects the interviewer's knowledge of individual diseases.

> **DOC:** Tell me about anything that seems to aggravate or bring these pains on.
> **PT:** Well, coffee does sometimes.
> **DOC:** What about aspirin, does that cause it? *[The interviewer would continue closed-endedly to ask about what she knows causes epigastric burning: other medications, tea, alcohol, tobacco, spicy foods.]*

DOC: (continuing after completing the above inquiry) Have you
noticed anything that helps, you know that relieves it?
PT: Eating almost anything, especially milk.
DOC: What about antacids?
PT: Yeah, they help a lot.

Often the patient is unable to describe moderating factors but can
say what he does (or avoids) during the symptoms; for example,
walk about, lie down, quit eating.

Associated Symptoms
It is uncommon to have only one symptom with an underlying
disease. Rather, there often are several symptoms specific to the
disease and, in addition, there may be secondary symptoms reflecting the general impact of the disease; for example, in a patient
with pneumonia, cough and chest pain are likely specific symptoms from the pneumonia while fatigue and irritability are nonspecific symptoms due to the general effect of the pneumonia on
the body. Associated symptoms are important because different
combinations have diagnostic importance; for example, in a patient
with weight loss, a good appetite often suggests diabetes mellitus
or hyperthyroidism while a poor appetite might suggest infection
or cancer.

The student detects associated symptoms by beginning open-
endedly, such as "Tell me any other symptoms that go along with
this." Closed-ended questions usually are required, however, as the
student pins down important details about the presence or absence
of symptoms that might be expected in association, as outlined in
Chapter 5; for example, in a patient with chest pain, one always
would want to know if they had shortness of breath.

DOC: Tell me any other symptoms that go with this burning pain.
PT: Well, a little diarrhea when it's bad. *[This new symptom and its
descriptors would be fully developed, just as we have done for the
epigastric burning pain.]*
DOC: Any other symptoms with it?
PT: Not really.
DOC: Any nausea? *[After the patient gives no additional symptoms, the interviewer uses her knowledge of common associations to make further specific inquiry, as expanded on in Chapter 5.]*

Summary

We use open- and closed-ended skills to establish a common, medical understanding of the individual symptom and then to refine it using seven descriptors, to enhance its diagnostic specificity. But individual symptoms are of little value in making a disease diagnosis. How to integrate multiple symptoms and describe the entire clinical problem in a way that points to an underlying disease are addressed in Chapter 5.

References

1. Barrows HS, Pickell GC. *Developing Clinical Problem-Solving Skills—A Guide to More Effective Diagnosis and Treatment*. New York: Norton Medical Books, 1991.
2. Platt FW. *Conversation Failure: Case Studies in Doctor-Patient Communication*. Tacoma, WA: Life Sciences Press, 1992.
3. Morgan WL, Engel GL. *The Clinical Approach to the Patient*. Philadelphia: Saunders, 1969.
4. Bates B. *A Guide to Physical Examination—and History Taking* (5th ed). Philadelphia: Lippincott, 1991.
5. Melzack R. *Pain Measurement and Assessment*. New York: Raven, 1983.

Doctor-Centered Process

This chapter describes, step by step, how the interviewer conducts the doctor-centered process. This involves the latter part of the History of the Present Illness (HPI) and Other Current Active Problems (OCAP), continuing directly from the patient-centered story, and the entire Health Issues (HI), Past Medical History (PMH), Social History (SH), Family History (FH), and Review of Systems (ROS).

The patient-centered process appropriately produced much raw information—the patient's personal experience of symptoms and his personal experience more generally. Most symptoms, however, require further clarification for diagnostic and therapeutic purposes. This requires that the interviewer take the lead to guide what becomes, by definition, a doctor-centered process. Although the interviewer assiduously avoided symptom-defining skills (Chapter 4) during the patient-centered process, in the doctor-centered process he actively uses these skills to synthesize raw patient-centered symptom data into a meaningful chronological story that identifies or suggests an underlying disease. The doctor-centered process also provides the extensive, routine data base needed by the interviewer. Nevertheless, the interviewer switches back to a patient-centered process when pertinent personal data or emotions arise, as they often do.

Recall our progress to this point. During the patient-centered process of the HPI (steps 1–5) the interviewer set the stage, obtained the chief complaint, established a flow of information, focused on the personal aspects of the data, and made a transition to the doctor-centered process of the HPI, the point where we now find ourselves. There are seven additional steps (steps 6–12) in the doctor-centered process to complete the interview, as outlined below. To illustrate each step, we will continue to follow Mrs. Jones.

Summary of the Interview to Put Current Doctor-Centered
Focus (italic) in Context

Patient-Centered Process for CC/HPI/OCAP
    Step 1—Setting the Stage
    Step 2—Agenda-Setting
    Step 3—Nonfocused Interviewing
    Step 4—Focused Interviewing
    Step 5—Transition to the Doctor-Centered Process

Doctor-Centered Process
    Step 6—HPI/OCAP—General Overview
    Step 7—HPI/OCAP—Chronological Description of All Primary
    and Secondary Data
    Step 8—Health Issues
    Step 9—Past Medical History
    Step 10—Social History
    Step 11—Family History
    Step 12—Review of Systems

Continuing the HPI/OCAP: General Overview (Step 6)

In many instances, a satisfactory overview will have occurred
during steps 2 through 4, in which case the interviewer summarizes and proceeds directly to step 7. If not, the overview is
developed at this point (see outline on pp. 78). An overview of the
major symptoms, when they began, and the most pressing current
issue are essential and require both open- and closed-ended skills.
The problem usually, but not always, will concern physical symptoms. In my example dialogue, I assume a physical focus with the
understanding that severe psychological symptoms also could be
addressed, as considered at the end of this discussion of the HPI. In
our continuing vignette of Mrs. Jones, the interviewer picks up at
the end of step 5 and completes an already initiated overview of her
problem.

Direct Continuation of Vignette of Mrs. Jones

(continued from end of Chapter 3 where student had already learned about Mrs. Jones' headache occurring in the context of a distressing work situation)

PT: Sure, that's what I came in for. *[To inquiry about changing the conversation to her headaches, cough, and colitis from the just ending patient-centered process]*

DOC: I know the headache is the biggest problem now. *[Starts generally and summarizes the primary physical complaint in an open-ended way and will shortly ask specific closed-ended questions for the details. If the interviewer somehow had not yet heard about the headache and other physical problems, he would now obtain a detailed description in the patient's own words. Ordinarily this will have occurred during the patient-centered process, as in Mrs. Jones' situation, and step 6 will be very brief.]*

PT: Yeah, it sure is.

DOC: When exactly did it begin? *[The interviewer wants to reaffirm the time frame of the headaches and uses a closed-ended question.]*

PT: Oh, just a few weeks after I got here. That's about 4 months ago now, so the headaches have been about 3 months.

DOC: When was the nausea? *[Pinning down this unknown detail with another closed-ended question]*

PT: Oh, that was later, a month or so after when they got worse.

DOC: And the colitis started in 1982 you said. How long has the cough been going on?

PT: Just the last couple weeks. *[The interviewer has now summarized Mrs. Jones' problems, established which is most important, and knows when each began. A good overview provides a general map of where to focus for details. Notice the increase in closed-ended questions and how they provide necessary details.]*

Continuing the HPI/OCAP: Chronological Description of All Primary and Secondary Data (Step 7)

Step 7 (see overview on page 78) is the most important and most difficult part of the doctor-centered process. The symptoms and secondary data that point to the patient's disease story will be further developed and clarified.

General Overview and Chronology of all HPI/OCAP Data

Step 6—General overview

Step 7—Chronological description of all primary and secondary data

1. Scanning and describing data without interpreting it
   a. Describing symptoms the patient presents
   b. Describing still-unmentioned symptoms in the already identified body system (or general health symptoms)
2. Interpreting data while obtaining it: testing hypotheses about the possible disease meaning of symptoms*

*Only clinical-level students are expected to be proficient with this style of inquiry.

As presented in Chapter 4, the interviewer converts each complaint to a symptom in the system review (ROS) and further identifies it according to the seven descriptors (location, quality, quantitation, chronology and timing, setting, moderating factors, and associated symptoms). But symptoms do not occur in isolation or at just one point in time. Introduced briefly in Chapter 4 (see associated symptoms, long-term course of symptoms), we now consider more extensively how to group symptoms and put all data in chronological order to serve as the database for eventually making a disease diagnosis.

Research has shown that students as well as seasoned clinicians make diagnoses of diseases by testing hypotheses during the course of the interview [1]. One first generates an hypothesis about a specific diagnosis, such as angina or migraine, and then deductively tests it by eliciting specific symptoms that do or do not support the hypothesized diagnosis [2]. Experts are faster, more efficient, and more accurate because of their greater knowledge and experience, which allows them to supplement their hypothesis-testing approach with pattern recognition and seasoned intuition [1].

Because of less experience and knowledge, preclinical and beginning clinical students are usually much less effective in making diagnoses by hypothesis-testing. To offset this, beginners often need to extensively scan patients for relevant symptoms and simply describe their findings without hypothesizing a diagnosis, an inductive process. Students then use these data to form hypotheses for subsequent testing (in a later interview), after having had time to read about the problems they have described. Beginning level students still test hypotheses during the interview but have this additional source of data from which they often can generate better and more hypotheses [2]. One scans only in relevant areas, does not ask the same questions of every patient, and does not simply elicit all known symptoms from the system review [2]. As students acquire clinical experience and their knowledge base grows, hypothesis-testing will become more prominent and scanning less so; nevertheless, even seasoned clinicians scan when hypothesis-testing is ineffective [2].

Preclinical and beginning clinical students can generate a surprisingly complete database with the purely "descriptive" or scanning approach first presented. We will then briefly consider how the student integrates the hypothesis-testing approach.

Scanning and Describing Data Without Interpreting It (For Preclinical and Beginning Clinical Students)

Symptoms and secondary data are grouped in two general categories: (1) data introduced by the patient, and (2) data not yet introduced that are in the same body system (as those already mentioned) or about general health.

Describing Symptoms the Patient Presents

The student begins with the most important problem to the patient and identifies all symptoms and secondary data starting from the beginning. Complaints are aggregated by common times of occurrence, translating each into a symptom as it arises and then refining the symptom using the seven descriptors. At times, it is easier to first obtain the patient's symptoms, and then fill in the secondary data. In either case, we make use of repeated queries for temporal connections such as, "Then what?" or "What happened after that?" or "And then?". The patient sometimes will not introduce secondary data and the interviewer must ask about treatment, procedures, diagnoses, and other secondary information. Alternatively, the patient may present a host of secondary data from which the student must sift out the symptoms.

The course of all data over time must be clearly understood. No time interval during the course of illness can be unaccounted for. Calendar dates and exact times are used when possible, always for recent or acute problems. More remote problems often can be marked by weeks, months, or even years.

As noted in the vignette below, closed-ended inquiry elicits most information. Periodic supportive remarks are appropriate, and a patient-centered atmosphere of warmth and understanding continues.

Continuation of Vignette of Mrs. Jones

PT: Just the last couple weeks.

DOC: Well, let's look more at the headaches when they began 3 months ago. *[Time of onset is already known. The student is starting at the beginning of the most important problem with a focused open-ended request.]*

PT: The headaches started one day at work, when I'd had a bad time with my boss. You know, that time I told you about. *[Mrs. Jones is referring to the earlier patient-centered process during which she told about the personal events associated with her headache. There is no need to go into this personal description again.]*

DOC: Tell me more of the features of the headache. *[A focused open-ended request which does not help much and the student proceeds to closed-ended inquiry.]*

PT: Well, like what?

DOC: You said it was in the right temple, can you point at it for me? Is it always in the same spot? *[The student is closed-endedly focusing away from the personal dimension and on the symptom itself, now getting the precise location.]*

PT: (puts hand over much of right side of head) It's all over here, sometimes larger than others. *[Sounds more diffuse than specifically in one location]*

DOC: Does it move anyplace else? *[Another of what will be many closed-ended questions as the student continues to develop the seven descriptors of illness. Note that the student is introducing new material into the conversation, appropriate for the doctor-centered process. The student also is leading the interaction.]*

PT: No, it stays right there. *[No radiation]*

DOC: Does it feel like inside your head or outside on the surface; you know, does it hurt to comb your hair or touch it?

PT: No, it doesn't hurt to touch it. It's down inside I think. *[A deep rather than superficial pain]*

DOC: Could you give me a description of what it feels like; you know, aching, burning, or however you'd describe it. *[It's appropriate to give examples, if necessary, as long as an answer is not suggested.]*

PT: Oh, it's more throbbing or pounding, like you feel each pulse beat. *[Quality of the pain identified, and no bizarre description]*

DOC: How do they begin, gradual or all of a sudden?

PT: Oh, pretty much out of the blue. *[Type of onset is sudden]*

DOC: How severe are they?

PT: Well, they're sometimes worse than having a baby! Especially when they get bad. And I've missed work a few days but not very often. *[Severe level of intensity at times and some disability]*

DOC: Wow, that's pretty bad. You've really had a lot of trouble with this! How long does each headache last, the shortest and the longest they might last? *[Empathic comments and behaviors are continued during the doctor-centered process]*

PT: At least a couple hours. When they get bad, they'll last up to 12 hours or so. *[Duration identified]*

DOC: What happens to the symptom during the time it's there?

PT: Well, it's not so bad at first but it just keeps getting worse and then the nausea comes. *[Course of individual symptom]*

DOC: How many do you have in a week or a month?

PT: I can have 2 or 3 a week when they're bad. You know every 2 to 3 days. *[Symptom frequency and intervals]*

DOC: How long have they been that often?

PT: Since things got bad in the last month, especially the last couple of weeks. Before that they were only once or twice a week. *[Total number can be calculated if important]*

DOC: Do you know of anything that brings them on? *[The student is not inquiring about the setting because he already knows that from the patient-centered process]*

PT: Well, just what I've told you, getting upset. Once or twice it seemed like having some wine did it but I was stressed then too. *[Perhaps another precipitant]*

DOC: Anything that worsens them once they've begun?

PT: No, they're bad enough already! Well, bright lights sure do, now that I think about it. *[An aggravating event identified]*

DOC: They sure have been bad. What seems to help them once they occur?

PT: Just lying down in a dark room, and an ice bag on my head. Well, the narcotic shot they gave me in the emergency room took it away too. *[Relief measures developed. Also, secondary data, the narcotic and the emergency room visit, are introduced by the patient.]*

DOC: What about the nausea? *[With a full description of the headache symptom, the student is moving now to better define an associated symptom, staying with primary data for the moment. Notice that a nonpain symptom has fewer appropriate descriptors; e.g., one usually does not try to identify location or radiation of nausea.]*

PT: That's when the headaches are bad.

DOC: Help me understand a little better what the nausea is like. *[A focused open-ended request]*

PT: Like I'm sick to my stomach and could vomit if it got worse. *[Quality of nausea]*

DOC: And how does it begin? *[A closed-ended question, as many of the subsequent inquiries will be]*

PT: Oh, it just kind of gradually comes on after the pain has been there awhile. *[Gradual onset]*

DOC: How bad is it, how severe?

PT: It's minor compared to the pain. It's never really been the problem the pain is. *[Not additionally severe or disabling]*

DOC: How often does the nausea occur?

PT: Just when the pain gets bad. I've probably had it each time with the headache in the month; that's when the pain has been worse. *[Number of episodes identified]*

DOC: You said this began about a month after the pain, so that means the nausea has been there about 2 months? *[Mrs. Jones has previously indicated the time of onset]*

PT: Yeah, but it's been worse in the last month.

DOC: How long does the nausea last once it begins?

PT: Oh, about a couple hours, when the headache finally goes away. *[Duration of nausea and relieving factor]*

DOC: Anything else that relieves it?

PT: Not that I know. I tried some antacid but it made me worse. *[Other aggravating and relieving factors explored]*

DOC: And what's the time between each episode?

PT: Same as the headaches, you know, every couple days. *[Intervals identified. Course of symptom and setting also can be inferred from what Mrs. Jones has said already since the nausea is linked to headaches.]*

DOC: Ever throw up with them?

PT: Just once. That's when I went to emergency. *[Associated symptom]*

DOC: How much did you vomit?

PT: Oh, just enough to soak a hankie. *[The student has obtained pertinent descriptions of the nausea and now has discovered another symptom, vomiting, which would now be similarly explored. Complicated patients, unlike Mrs. Jones, can take considerable time in obtaining appropriate details of each symptom.]*

DOC/PT: *[Not recounted here, the student and patient now develop details of the patient's vomiting. As students gain experience, they will recognize that the headache, nausea, and vomiting go together. This allows them to develop the symptoms simultaneously, as shown next, and avoid the repetition that is noted above.]*

DOC: It sounds like you went to emergency once when it was bad. What's been the course of the headaches and nausea; you know better, worse, or about the same?

PT: They are getting worse. They last longer and more often in the last 2 weeks. *[The overall course of the primary data is learned]*

DOC: Who've you seen for them? *[A good description of symptoms and their course to the present has been obtained and the student is beginning to move away from symptoms to associated secondary data.]*

PT: Nobody, except the emergency room a week ago. I thought the aspirin would help.

DOC: Have you taken anything else?

PT: Nothing except that one shot; a narcotic of some sort I think.

DOC: Did they do any tests on you in the emergency room?

PT: Yeah, they did a blood count and a urine test.

DOC: No scans or any other types of x-rays of your head? *[Recent inquiry is aimed at understanding pertinent secondary data. Notice the repeated use of closed-ended questions to obtain a more precise description of the symptoms.]*

PT: No.

Describing Still Unmentioned Symptoms in the Already Identified Body System (or General Health Symptoms)

To this point, the interviewer has addressed symptoms volunteered by the patient (and related secondary data). But there often are other pertinent symptoms, either by their presence or absence; the absence of a symptom can be just as important diagnostically as its presence. The student thus needs to develop a more complete profile of the patient's problem.

Other pertinent data are the presence or absence of other symptoms in the body system already identified as symptomatic. We can often assume that symptoms in the same system are related to the same underlying disease process. One knows what the patient's major complaints are and can therefore identify the body system of likely disease involvement from the system review; for example, hesitancy and increased urinary frequency suggest that the urinary system is affected by some disease. At times, however, a symptom can suggest more than one system as a source of disease; for example, substernal pain reflecting disease in the gastrointestinal system (esophagitis) or the cardiopulmonary system (angina). When there is any question, both systems are considered as possible areas of involvement.

Using closed-ended inquiry, the student determines the presence or absence of each symptom possibility in the system(s) involved. In the two examples above, inquiry about all other possible urinary symptoms would occur in the first instance (dysuria, bloody urine, particulate matter in the urine, and so on until all possible urinary symptoms in the system review had been screened), and inquiry about all possible cardiopulmonary and gastrointestinal symptoms would take place in the second (hemoptysis, orthopnea, vomiting, diarrhea, and so on).

Inquiry often reveals the presence of symptoms the patient has forgotten or not thought important, and can at times provide crucial diagnostic information; for example, in the above patient with urinary complaints, discovering the periodic presence of particulate matter in the urine in association with bloody urine might suggest renal calculi. Frequently, however, this inquiry indicates the absence of most symptoms on the list, a fact of diagnostic importance; for example, the absence of hematuria in this patient weighs against renal calculi as well as serious bladder or renal diseases.

Inquiring about symptoms of general health (see the System Review in Chap. 4) fills out the symptom profile. Inquiry about appetite, weight, general feeling of well-being, pain, and fever is germane in most patients, whatever system their symptoms reside in. Many diseases, especially more serious ones, exhibit one or more of these symptoms. In our vignette, predominantly closed-ended inquiry continues to be relied on, and supportive remarks continue to be interspersed.

Continuation of Vignette of Mrs. Jones

DOC: Any other symptoms you might have had? *[A focused, open-ended request, phrased as a question]*

PT: Well, nothing that I think of.

DOC: Ever had problems with dizziness or light-headedness? *[Because the patient's major symptom, headaches, is a neuropsychiatric system symptom, the student is beginning to closed-endedly inquire about other possible symptoms in the neuropsychiatric system.]*

PT: Not now. I used to get carsick as a kid and did a couple times then.

DOC: Ever had a fainting spell?

PT: No.

DOC: Stiff neck?

PT: No.

DOC: Any problems with the vision?

PT: No. I don't even use glasses.

DOC: Any double vision?

PT: No.

DOC: Difficulty hearing?

PT: No.

DOC: Any change in your sense of taste or smell?

PT: No.

DOC: Any pain in the face?

PT: No. *[The student would continue exploring all remaining symptoms in the neuropsychiatric system: facial paralysis; difficulty swallowing or with speech; difficulty elevating the shoulders; muscle weakness or movement difficulty; extremity numbness, tingling, decreased sensation, or paralysis; the shakes or tremor; difficulty with balance or walking; seizures; peculiar thoughts or perceptions; depression or anxiety; difficulties with memory, orientation, judgment, attention, or concentration; insomnia, excessive sleepiness, or nightmares; anhedonia.]*

DOC: Besides the nausea and vomiting once, have you had any other digestive problems? *[A focused, open-ended question starts a new area of inquiry. The student will now obtain a complete profile of the patient's other major symptom, nausea.]*

PT: There haven't been any.

DOC: *[Even though the patient indicates none was present, the student would now closed-endedly go through the symp-*

toms in the gastrointestinal system not already addressed: appetite, weight, heartburn, abdominal pain, vomiting blood (hematemesis), bloody or black stools, constipation or diarrhea, dark urine or jaundice, and rectal pain or excessive gas. The student then shifts to general symptoms.]

DOC: You've told me a lot already about this, but how've you been in general? *[A focused open-ended question introduces a new area of inquiry, her general health. Information about appetite and weight will already have been obtained during the above inquiry about gastrointestinal symptoms.]*

PT: Great, except all these things.

DOC: What do you enjoy in your life, you know for recreation or fun? *[Another focused open-ended question for information about general health.]*

PT: Well, my painting is my true love. I like to do that every day, come rain or shine. It really helps get my mind off of things. *[Active outside interests weigh against anhedonia and its frequent concomitant, depression.]*

DOC: That's great. I'm impressed how you do so many things. Any problem with fevers or chills? *[The student continues to make supportive comments and asks a closed-ended question.]*

PT: No. *[Therefore, there is no problem with general health symptoms of appetite, weight, fever, chills, or anhedonia.]*

Interpreting Data While Obtaining It: Testing Hypotheses About the Possible Disease Meaning of Symptoms (For Clinical Students and Graduates)

The preclinical student now has a complete profile and chronology of symptoms although they have not been interpreted or grouped in a way that points to specific diseases that could cause them. Just recounting symptoms usually does not identify a disease. Nor has the preclinical interviewer accounted for potentially significant symptoms in other systems. Moreover, simply inquiring about all symptoms outside the involved system is not feasible, would take too long, is intellectually unsound, and is boring [2].

It may be necessary initially for the beginning clinical student to obtain much data by the scanning or descriptive approach. To increase the diagnostic value of the interview, however, the student must learn to actively test hypotheses during the interview. This requires bringing to the bedside a knowledge of diseases and their unique symptom constellations and other diagnostic features, learned from standard textbooks. Chest pain, for example, has well over 20 possible disease causes, each with unique symptom and other diagnostic features and, often, different associated symptoms (e.g., angina pectoris, myocardial infarction, esophagitis, pneumonia, rib fracture, pulmonary embolus, or pericarditis).

How does the interviewer test hypotheses during the interview? Based on unique symptom characteristics and secondary data suggesting one diagnosis over the others, and on knowledge of what diseases are most common, the interviewer ranks disease possibilities in his mind starting very early in the interview [1–3]. The interviewer then seeks additional diagnostic data (primary and secondary) to support the current best choice; if data have already been obtained descriptively, these new data will be largely outside the involved system. If not supported, another disease hypothesis becomes the best choice to explain the symptom(s) and is similarly explored. By following this process of testing multiple, ever-changing hypotheses, one eventually arrives at the best diagnostic possibility. It is not uncommon, for example, to start with one disease hypothesis (angina) and, based on symptom descriptors and associated symptoms, end with a quite different one (esophagitis). For example, because of substernal chest pain radiating into the arms, the student's first hypothesis was angina. But, he knew esophagitis also was a possible cause of chest pain radiating to the arms and asked about descriptors and other symptoms associated with this diagnosis and they were present (precipitation of pain by coffee; relief by belching and antacids; poor appetite) and other descriptors expected with angina were not present (no relationship of pain to exertion). When a hypothesis is well supported, it becomes a "diagnosis." A diagnosis can derive from the history alone (e.g., angina) but sometimes additional data from the physical examination (e.g., enlarged liver) or the laboratory (e.g., low hemoglobin) are needed before one can establish a diagnosis [2].

The more knowledge and experience, the more facile and efficient one becomes in formulating the diagnosis and knowing the proper questions to ask during an interview, rather than in a subsequent interview. Nevertheless, virtually all beginning clinical students will find themselves fully synthesizing the diagnosis only after the interview—when they have read about the problem, talked again with the patient to clarify issues they overlooked, and discussed the problem with faculty and residents. Although this vast topic of clinical diagnostics [1–6] is outside the province of this text, the process of clinical problem-solving is illustrated in the example below. This shows how the student tests hypotheses while obtaining the HPI.

An Example of Clinical Problem-Solving

Clinicians proceed, much as Sherlock Holmes [2], by first obtaining a few bits of presenting data (e.g., nonradiating chest pain, fever, shortness of breath, and a swollen leg in a 70-year-old man) with which to generate the current best hypothesis (e.g., pulmonary embolus) and then ask specific questions (e.g., hemoptysis, which means coughing up blood) that would further support or detract from this hypothesis [1–3]. In this example, the clinician introduces the previously unmentioned hemoptysis because her first hypothesis was pulmonary embolus and this symptom is pertinent to its diagnosis. Let us say that hemoptysis was not present but the clinician pursued the hypothesis further by inquiring if the leg swelling was recent or if there had been any immobility of the leg recently, common findings of some diagnostic value in pulmonary embolism. We'll suppose that symptoms began following a 12-hour car ride just 3 days ago and that the clinician became more confident of pulmonary embolus as a possible diagnosis.

The interviewer, however, tests alternative hypotheses among the other most likely diseases causing this patient's chest pain. For example, the advanced student also would consider distinguishing questions supporting myocardial infarction (substernal location of pain, crushing pain, diaphoresis), pneumonia (fever, cough, chills), rib fracture (injury), pericarditis (pain relieved by sitting up and leaning forward, and aggravated by lying supine), lung cancer (weight loss, cigarette or asbestos exposure), and a host of other possibilities as long as they reflected reasonable possible causes of the patient's chest pain and other symptoms. Notice that none of these symptoms had been mentioned to this point, that the clinician introduced them closed-endedly, that if left to routine inquiry many would have been completely dissociated from the HPI (chest trauma and cigarette use are asked about in the PMH usually), and that some may never have arisen without such hypothesis-driven inquiry (relief of pain from sitting up is not a routine question).

The clinician in this case would of course proceed to obtain a complete history and physical examination and appropriate laboratory data to clarify her hypotheses and, hopefully, establish a diagnosis.

Continuation of Vignette of Mrs. Jones

DOC: Ever had problems with swelling or pains in the joints? *[The student has the hypothesis that vasculitis might be causing headache and knows that it is sometimes associated with arthritis. He is thus inquiring closed-endedly about specific primary data outside the system involved to support this hypothesis.]*

PT: No.

DOC: Ever had any dancing or bright, shimmering lights in your vision with the headaches? *[The student knows that this symptom (scintillating scotomata) is of diagnostic value in migraine and is properly inquiring specifically about it as a way to build support for the hypothesis of migraine headaches.]*

PT: No.

DOC: Because these could be vascular headaches, you know like migraine, I need to ask you some specifics about that. Do you use birth control pills or other hormones? *[The student is beginning to formulate diagnostic hypotheses about what has caused the headaches. He suspects migraine from the clinical story. Accordingly, it is appropriate to obtain additional supporting diagnostic data and, hence, the question about birth control pills. In addition, because head injuries also can cause headaches, the student will ask about that as an alternative hypothesis. Indeed, any possible causes that have been entertained could be further addressed in this way; for example, if the student were suspicious of meningitis from the story, perhaps because of intermittent fever and stiff neck, additional questions to support or refute that hypothesis would be in order: any rashes, exposure, and whatever else the student considered important in supporting a diagnosis of meningitis.]*

PT: Yeah, I've been on them for the last 6 years. *[The student would pursue the type, dosage, and experience with this later in the PMH—although could do so now also.]*

DOC: Any family history of migraine? *[Because a positive family history supports the hypothesis of migraine, these questions are included here rather than in the FH.]*

PT: One of my aunts had what they called "sick headaches" when she was young but they all cleared up when she got a lot older.

DOC: By the way, have you ever had any head injuries? *[The* *student is testing a nonmigraine hypothesis for the head-ache.]*

PT: No.

DOC: Have you ever been unconscious for any reason?

PT: No.

DOC: Any neck injuries or problems there? *[Neck problems also can cause headaches and the student is exploring this hypothesis.]*

PT: Nope.

DOC: Well, we need to change to some other questions now, about your colitis, cough, and past medical history, if you feel finished talking about this. Anything else we need to cover, before we go on? *[It continues to be important to mention transitions, check if the patient is finished, and see if she or he has anything further to add to the topic at hand.]*

PT: That's fine. You've covered everything, I think. *[This evaluation by a beginning clinical level student shows how the new interviewer first obtains data in the involved system to help develop hypotheses, and then tests the hypotheses with selective questions designed to support or refute them.]*

Procedural Issues

When more than one problem has been raised, the student evaluates it in the same way. For example, Mrs. Jones also had colitis and a recent cough. These now could be systematically explored. If these are not currently active health problems, though, they also can be explored as part of the PMH. And when not contributing to current problems, as in Mrs. Jones' situation, they are included in the PMH portion of the written report. When they are contributing to current problems, they are included as OCAP at the end of the HPI.

This is a lot for the student to assimilate, and to do so requires much practice. It is reassuring that, once the symptoms in the system review and the symptom-defining skills are learned in their clinical context, this process becomes quite reflexive. Nor does it take the seasoned clinician long. Most can conduct a full HPI/OCAP, HI, PMH, SH, FH, and ROS with a patient like Mrs. Jones in 30 to 40 minutes. With advancing skills and knowledge of diseases, the student learns which are the most pertinent questions and how to ask them efficiently. (See the end of Chapter 6 for a discussion of how much time the beginning clinical student will need to spend with the patient.)

Much of the interview occurs by predominantly closed-ended inquiry, which raises two important issues. First, poorly conducted closed-ended inquiry can lead to considerable bias of the data. Suggestions for minimizing bias in closed-ended inquiry are listed below:

---

1. Proceed from general to specific—Start with an open-ended question in each major area.
2. Use single questions—Avoid questions like "Have you ever had headaches, fainting, loss of vision, blurred vision, poor memory, or a stroke?" Rather, one might ask, "Have you ever had headaches?"
3. Don't suggest a response by the way the question is framed—Avoid "You haven't had any blood in the urine, have you?"
4. Give equal weight to alternative answers—Advise "It sounds like there is some pain with exertion, but what about when you're not exerting?"
5. Don't interpret data while collecting it—Avoid "Must be hemorrhoids. Ever had any nausea or vomiting?"
6. Give balanced attention to all aspects—Advise "We've talked a lot about your constipation, but not much yet about the chest pain."
7. Don't confuse the patient with rapid shifts or technical language—Avoid "Did they do an ERCP or another endoscopy; were any lesions found?"
8. Ensure that the conversation is congruent with the patient's experience—Advise in appropriate situation "Does the sore spot ever flake off, like peeling paint?"

Adapted from Morgan WL, Engel GL. *The Clinical Approach to the Patient*. Philadelphia: Saunders, 1969, and Enelow AJ, Swisher SN. *Interviewing and Patient Care* (3rd ed.). New York: Oxford University Press, 1986.

Second, because we are in the doctor-centered process, one can ask direct questions that insert new information into the conversation where necessary. This is especially helpful in testing hypotheses; for example, in a patient with a chronic cough, it is perfectly appropriate to introduce this material: "Are you a cigarette smoker?" or "Have you lost weight?"

The HPI/OCAP concludes when all presenting symptoms have been addressed. The clinician, although perhaps not the beginning clinical student, understands the problem and has the best possible disease explanation in mind if not the actual diagnosis. Interviewers also more fully recognize the close interaction of symptoms and secondary data with the personal data obtained during the patient-centered process.

The student makes a statement about changing the conversation to some material "we haven't yet covered about your past medical history," as done with Mrs. Jones above. One inquires if the patient thinks his story has been completely discussed, summarizes, and asks if the patient has anything further to add.

Addressing a Predominantly Psychological Problem

In patients with psychiatric diseases or other serious psychological problems, the personal contextual data obtained during the patient-centered process usually are not sufficient for complete evaluation. Steps 1 through 5 are just the beginning. In the doctor-centered HPI, the interviewer pins down details about the psychological problem, just as one would with any other disease problem. One elicits the patient's symptoms and tests hypotheses about the underlying diagnosis by selectively testing different diagnostic possibilities. For example, depression in a patient may have been apparent during steps 1 through 5, but it now is the interviewer's task to explore its possible disease causes, potential complications, and treatment options. Using scanning open-ended inquiry followed by closed-ended inquiry one differentiates, for example, major depression, bipolar disorder, schizophrenia, drugs, and medical diseases as causes of the depression. Just as the student gains more experience with the diagnosis of medical diseases during clinical rotations, he will learn much more about psychological diagnoses during psychiatry rotations.

On the other hand, many medical patients are like Mrs. Jones and have no apparent overriding psychological problem or diagnosis. Does that statement surprise you after all we have heard about Mrs. Jones' job stresses and interpersonal conflicts? While important to the student to understand the patient, such conflict does not necessarily bespeak disease. Indeed, this type of problem defines our personal lives and is not outside the realm of normal experience. Additional personal details for patients like Mrs. Jones usually are obtained in the SH.

Health Issues (Step 8)

Health issues (HI) are important information often omitted from the database but nonetheless essential to best understand and help the patient. Health issues are problems in the following areas: ethical-social-spiritual issues, functional status, health-promoting and health-maintenance habits, and potential health hazards [7–10].

Each major HI area in the outline below is initiated with a focused open-ended request or question ("Tell me what you do to stay healthy"), which is followed with enough closed-ended questions to get the necessary details. Because health issues concern many sensitive areas, the student is especially careful to be patient, courteous, and understanding to ensure continuation of the patient-centered atmosphere. Patients are reassured that the questions are routine and asked of everyone. Tension-laden areas are addressed delicately with considerable use of open-ended and emotion-handling skills; that is, one may need to resume the patient-centered process described earlier. The interviewing strategy for obtaining very sensitive material (e.g., sexual or drug abuse history), is expanded upon in Chapter 6.

Health Issues (Step 8)*
1. Ethical-social-spiritual issues: advance directives, power of attorney, whom to contact if the patient cannot speak for her/himself, and spiritual practices
2. Functional status: dressing, bathing, feeding, transferring, walking, shopping, using the toilet, using a telephone, cooking, cleaning, driving, taking medications, managing finances, and cognitive function; extent of interference with normal life
3. Health-promoting and health-maintenance activities
    a. Health-promoting habits: diet, seat belts, using helmet with bicycle or motorcycle, protection of self and others from poisonous substances (including medications) and dangerous circumstances at home and at work, exercise, relaxation, recreation
    b. Health screening: periodic health exams, mammograms, Pap smear, sigmoidoscopy, stools for occult blood, cholesterol, blood sugar, serologic test for syphilis, tuberculosis skin testing, HIV testing, prostatic evaluation, dental

    check-up, audiograms, eye exam, tonometry; self-exam-
    ination (breasts, genitals, and skin)
  c. Disease prophylaxis: diphtheria, pertussis, tetanus, polio,
      measles, German measles, hepatitis, influenza, vaccine for
      pneumococcal pneumonia, for diseases in areas of foreign
      travel
4. Health hazards
  a. Use of addicting substances: caffeine, tobacco, alcohol,
      street drugs, prescription medications
  b. Sexual practices: activity, preferences, diseases, abuse,
      risky habits, contraception, satisfaction
  c. Abuse: sexual, physical, verbal, psychological, other

*Adapted from Platt FW. *Conversation Repair*. Boston: Little, Brown, 1995, and Kuhn
CC. A spiritual inventory of the medically ill patient. *Psychiatr Med* 6:87–100, 1988.

Ethical-Social-Spiritual Issues

The student needs to inquire about advance directives (e.g., "do
not resuscitate" wishes, living will, use of a respirator to sustain
life), power of attorney, and whom to contact in the event of serious
health problems, especially in the severely ill, disabled, and elderly.
These data are essential for any patient who may become seriously
ill and unable to speak for himself.

Rarely addressed but essential information, especially in times
of crisis, are the patient's spiritual affiliations and beliefs, whether
attached to a formal religion or not. The student tries to understand
what is ultimately meaningful for patients, how this relates to their
suffering, what their belief and faith is, who and what they love,
their meditation or prayer practices, their orientation to giving and
forgiving, and the patients' actual worship practices; that is, the
integration of mind, body, and spirit [8].

Functional Status
Especially in the elderly and those with disabling problems, it is
necessary that the student know what the patient's functional
status is; for example, how well they can dress themselves, walk,
shop, use the toilet, and keep track of their bank account. In
addition, one needs to make an assessment of how much a disability interferes with the patient's life and wishes; for example, one

may no longer be able to climb stairs but this does not interfere with what the patient wants to do or, alternatively, the same disability works a great hardship by preventing the patient from attending baseball games.

Health-Promoting and Health-Maintenance Habits

The student asks what the patient thinks of her own health status and then inquires specifically about health-promoting habits. Does the patient partake of low-salt and low-fat diet with healthy protein and calorie content; use a seat belt and have airbags; use a helmet while riding a bicycle or motorcycle; have weapons in the home safely stored; have a smoke detector; have all poisonous substances (including medications) safe from childrens' reach; have safe-guards against toxic exposure and dangerous situations at home and at work; exercise at least three times weekly; take satisfactory amounts of time for relaxation, and enjoy outside recreational activities?

There also are a number of recommended health-screening procedures (which vary by age, circumstance, and gender) that the student will want to ensure are up-to-date: periodic health exam-ination, mammograms, Pap smear, sigmoidoscopy, stools for oc-cult blood, cholesterol, blood sugar, serologic test for syphilis, tuberculosis skin testing, HIV testing, prostatic evaluation, dental check, audiograms, eye exam, and tonometry. It also is important to know if patients are performing self-examination of the breasts, testes, penis, and skin; a significant disease often can be detected early when a patient is more amenable to treatment.

Finally, one determines the patient's level of disease prophylaxis: diphtheria, pertussis, tetanus, polio, measles, German measles, hepatitis, influenza, pneumococcal pneumonia, and diseases unique to areas of intended foreign travel.

Health Hazards

Use of Addicting Substances

Patients often minimize this material, particularly drug or alco-hol usage, and inquiry produces tension for the student and patient alike. The student asks about duration, amount, and type of addict-ing substance used; for example, drinks three beers daily except six or seven per day on weekends, and started this 11 years ago; smoked two packages of cigarettes daily for 8 years. Data about alcohol problems can be obtained using the CAGE questionnaire.

CAGE is an acronym for the four highlighted areas: (1) Have you ever tried to Cut down? (2) Do you get Angry when people talk to you about your drinking? (3) Do you feel Guilty about your drinking? and (4) Do you ever take an Eye opener? [11]. In addition, the student inquires if the patient has had problems from using addicting substances (divorce, job loss, delirium tremens with alcohol withdrawal, emphysema from cigarettes), attempted to quit or decrease the habit, why he was or wasn't successful in stopping, and if she is interested in getting help abstaining. Problems with the legal system, with sharing drug equipment, and with other substance abuse problems in the patient's life also are essential data. Finally, particularly with drug and alcohol abuse, the interviewer looks for the psychiatric issues that commonly attend these problems (e.g., anxiety, depression). Indeed, full primary and secondary data are elicited for any perceived drug or alcohol problem. When alcohol or drug abuse exists, it often belongs in the HPI because it frequently relates to the major problem the patient has and almost always has a major impact on the patient's health. Students will learn the details of psychiatric interviewing and evaluation of drug and alcohol abuse during clinical work.

Sexual Practices

Although sexual activity per se is of course not hazardous, many hazardous situations occur as a result of patients' sexual habits [12]. A good history requires the following information: heterosexual, homosexual, or bisexual orientation; current sexual activity (type, amount, and number of partners); past sexual activity (type, amount, and number of partners); risky sexual habits; condom usage; sexual satisfaction and pleasure; contraceptive measures; sexually transmitted diseases; impotence; nonorgasmic; and any other sexual concerns. Where sexual disorder is prominent, attendant psychiatric disease, such as depression and anxiety, is common and must be clarified. The history is not complete until the student also learns about the patient's relationship with a partner(s), especially their communication patterns.

Abuse

Abuse is increasingly prominent in many areas of patients' lives, and the student inquires specifically about sexual abuse, physical abuse, verbal abuse, and psychological abuse. All patients are potential recipients or perpetrators, and the extent of abuse may vary from frequent and severe to infrequent and mild. Particularly susceptible have been women, children, and the elderly. Such stories are quite common in those with both medical and psychological illnesses.

Because obtaining all HI items is a time-consuming task, graduates and advanced clinical level students may not obtain all of them at the first visit, completing them instead over time. Beginning clinical level students, however, are advised to initially obtain complete information in all areas as a way of learning the categories and beginning to appreciate the rich diversity of patients.

Continuation of Vignette with Mrs. Jones

DOC: Let me ask you some other questions about what you do to stay healthy. *[A good open-ended start into health issues. Because of space constraints, we will again simply summarize the findings about Mrs. Jones, some of which required return to a patient-centered process of inquiry. She has done nothing about advance directives but thinks they are a good idea. Her church attendance has been flagging since moving here due to her busy schedule. She has no functional limitations. We know about her work but also learn that she worries about being a "workaholic" and not taking enough time for her painting, which, it turns out, she doesn't do every day. She and her husband socialize frequently. She is trying to be a good model for her "lax husband" and always uses her seat belt, exercises three times weekly in a 45-minute aerobics class, maintains her weight around 120 pounds, and follows a low-fat/low-salt diet. She wants to do more about better relaxing but isn't sure what to do. She has yearly Pap smears and performs breast self-examination about a week after each menstrual period. She had her "baby shots" years ago and had a tetanus shot 2 years ago when she punctured her hand with a nail. Except for an occasional cup of coffee and glass of wine, she has never used addicting substances. She has been satisfied with her sexual life until the last 3 months when she has had less interest in sexual intercourse (now reduced from three or four times weekly to once weekly) and her husband has had inconstant difficulties with impotence; she has no reason to suspect her husband is not monogamous. She thinks the sexual problem "will take care of itself" when her job problems are resolved. She's not interested in talking any further about it at this point. She's had only two other sexual partners, prior to marriage. There's no history of sexually transmitted disease or sexual abuse (or other types of abuse now or in the past), and she and her husband are heterosexual.]*

Past Medical History (Step 9)

The past medical history (PMH) elicits information about significant past medical events [9,10]. Events occurring in the past that are related to the HPI/OCAP, however, are elicited as part of the HPI/OCAP. For instance, in a patient presenting with chest pain, the prior history of myocardial infarction usually is obtained in the HPI rather than the PMH. Similarly, because of the close association of diabetes and coronary artery disease, if this patient also were a diabetic of 20 years duration, those data would be elicited in the HPI. On the other hand, if the same patient presented with diverticulitis or hip fracture, the cardiovascular history would be obtained in the PMH as long as it was not an active problem. These distinctions aren't always clear, and there is no rigid right or wrong about where one places or where one obtains historical data. And, of course, one sometimes elicits data pertinent to the HPI while obtaining the PMH; it is relocated to the HPI when being written up or presented.

Similar approaches used with the doctor-centered process of the HPI/OCAP elicit the PMH. Each major area is shown below and is addressed with a focused, open-ended screening question; for example, "Tell me about any previous hospitalizations" (any other medical problems, any surgeries). This is followed with enough closed-ended questions to get the necessary details for all items mentioned. Simple closed-ended inquiry suffices in obtaining much data within these categories ("Ever had any broken bones?").

Past Medical History (PMH) (Step 9)*
1. Hospitalizations: surgical, nonsurgical, psychiatric, obstetric, rehabilitation, other
2. Other medical, surgical, or psychological problems: childhood illnesses, injuries, accidents, illnesses, unexplained problems, procedures, tests, psychotherapy, other
3. Screen for major diseases: rheumatic fever, diabetes mellitus, tuberculosis, venereal diseases, cancer, heart attack, stroke; and major treatments in the past (cortisone, blood transfu-

sions, insulin, digitalis, anticoagulants); and visits to the doctor during the last year

4. Medications and other treatments: prescribed, over the counter, alternative therapies and health care, and "nonmedications" (laxatives, tonics, hormones, birth control pills, vitamins)

5. Allergies and drug reactions: allergic diseases (e.g., asthma, hay fever), drugs, foods, environmental

6. Menstrual and obstetric history (for women): onset of menses, duration, cycle length, discomfort, number of pads daily, birth control pills and other hormonal preparations, pregnancies, abortions (spontaneous), abortions (induced), deliveries of living children, other deliveries, complications of pregnancy, menopause

---

*Adapted from Morgan WL, Engel GL. *The Clinical Approach to the Patient*. Philadelphia: Saunders, 1969; and Billings AJ, Stoeckle JD. *The Clinical Encounter: A Guide to the Medical Interview and Case Presentation*. Chicago: Year Book, 1989.

The student continues to support the patient and ensure a patient-centered atmosphere. Inquiring periodically how the patient is responding to the interview itself helps. It can be tiring, confusing, and even upsetting. For example, one almost always reassures patients that certain questions do not reflect suspicion but, rather, are routinely asked of everyone; for example, regarding cancer, diabetes mellitus, or memory loss.

We now will expand upon the PMH outline. When a problem with significance for the patient's health is found in any areas listed, the student reviews the symptoms and makes his own diagnosis, often requiring outside records to be certain. For serious or current problems, one cannot accept as final a patient's understanding of diagnoses or interpretations of treatments. The interviewer follows the already described procedure: converts complaints to symptoms in the system review and refines them with the seven descriptors, and then orders relevant primary data (symptoms) and secondary data (doctors, hospitals, tests) into chronological sequence.

For PMH problems with little significance to present health (appendectomy or tonsillectomy many years ago), little detail is needed other than getting the patient's version of diagnosis, complications, and statement that there have been no subsequent problems. Indeed, time constraints and the patient's comfort discourage acquiring unnecessary data.

One identifies significant past problems by inquiring in the following areas (outlined above).

Hospitalizations
Hospitalizations may identify the most serious problems the patient has experienced: surgical, nonsurgical, psychiatric, obstetric, rehabilitative, and any other type. The more recent and the more serious a hospitalization, the more data are required, sometimes more extensive than the HPI; for example, in a patient who is admitted with a hip fracture as the primary problem but who had a history of three heart attacks, the student would need to elicit extensive details of all primary and secondary cardiovascular data. Hospitalizations usually are obtained in chronological order.

Other Medical, Surgical, or Psychological Problems
Here one seeks significant past problems by specific inquiry about childhood illnesses (e.g., measles, mumps, German measles, chicken pox), injuries, accidents, illnesses requiring several visits, unexplained problems, procedures, tests, and psychotherapy.

Screen for Major Diseases
To screen for problems that might not yet have been identified, one makes specific inquiry, for example, about diabetes, tuberculosis, venereal diseases, rheumatic fever, heart attacks, strokes, or cancer. Similarly, the student asks about prior treatment that suggests serious problems: cortisone, insulin, blood transfusions, digitalis, and anticoagulants. Finally, the student inquires about all health visits to the doctor or others during the last year.

Medications and Other Treatments
Prescribed and other medications are listed with dose, duration of use, reason for use, and any adverse reactions. One also obtains a list of medications used during the last year that are not presently being taken. Specific inquiry about agents sometimes not considered to be medications is necessary as well: laxatives, tonics, hormones, birth control pills, and vitamins. Inquiry also is made about agents obtained over-the-counter, from alternative healers, or from other sources such as a friend. In all instances the student identifies the contents, often requiring that the pharmacy be contacted or that the patient bring in the actual medications so that they can be definitively identified, particularly when all the patient knows is that "I'm taking a brown pill for my circulation." Some-

times it helps to consult the Physicians' Desk Reference, which has color photographs of many commonly used brand-name medications [13].

The student asks about nonpharmacologic forms of treatment, whether administered by self or others, including physical therapy, biofeedback, relaxation techniques, yoga, acupuncture, psychotherapy of any type (e.g., individual, group), diet, and exercise. One specifically inquires about so-called alternative methods of treatment (e.g., homeopathy, herbal medicine, chiropractic) since these often are not mentioned out of embarrassment or fear of angering the physician [14].

Allergies and Drug Reactions
If not already ascertained, one asks about asthma, hay fever, hives, and atopic eczema because these are common allergic disorders; asthma has nonallergic dimensions as well. Such patients also may be more sensitive to certain medications (e.g., aspirin in asthmatics).

Drug reactions can be allergic/immunologic (rash due to penicillin) or nonimmunologic (candida vaginitis due to an antibiotic). Patients seldom make this distinction but the interviewer must because allergic reactions usually militate against subsequent use of the medication while alterations in dosage and frequency can sometimes allow later use following a nonallergic drug reaction. One lists all allergic or other drug reactions, dose and duration of use of the agent, specific symptoms (e.g., hives, anaphylaxis, rash) and secondary data (e.g., desensitization, skin tests, cortisone), recurrence, history of reexposure, and final outcome.

Menstrual and Obstetric History (for Women)
Essential information to obtain from women and girls about menses is age at onset, duration, cycle length, discomfort, and number of tampons or pads daily. Use of birth control pills or other hormonal preparations also is sometimes elicited here. Obstetric histories include number of pregnancies, spontaneous abortions, induced abortions, deliveries of living children and their outcome, other deliveries and reason for adverse outcome, and any complications of pregnancy. Menopausal problems also can be elicited here. The menstrual/obstetric history often is elicited in the HPI when genitourinary problems are the focus.

We now pick up again with Mrs. Jones.

Continuation of Vignette of Mrs. Jones

DOC: Tell me about any hospitalizations you've had, you know, other than that time for the colitis. *[Although not recounted in the doctor-centered HPI/OCAP or PMH, for space considerations, the student already has addressed Mrs. Jones' colitis and cough; the results of this inquiry are given in the write-up in Appendix B.]*

PT: I had my tonsils out as a kid.

DOC: Any other hospitalizations? *[The student might have asked why the tonsillectomy was done, and about any complications or subsequent problems.]*

PT: Well, I did break my arm once in high school and they had to set it.

DOC: How's that been since? Any problem? *[It would be important to know how it was broken.]*

PT: No, it's just fine. I play tennis and have no trouble.

DOC/PT: Other hospitalizations (no), injuries (no), accidents (no), or sickness (no)? *[These questions are asked and answered individually.]*

DOC: Didn't you mention having kids?

PT: Oh, yeah. I forgot! They're 6 and 8. But I had no trouble delivering. *[This sounds uncomplicated at this point and the student will get the details of the menstrual and obstetric history at the end of the PMH although it could just as easily be done now.]*

DOC/PT: I'm going to give you some specific diseases now and just tell me if you've ever had them (By the way, these are routine questions; I'm not asking because I suspect something): rheumatic fever (no), scarlet fever (no), diabetes (no), TB (no), sexually transmitted diseases (no), cancer (no), stroke (no), heart attack (no), or any other diseases (no). *[In a series of questions like this, each one is asked individually and the patient allowed sufficient time to answer; the patient should not feel pressured nor should a whole string of questions be asked at once. It is important throughout to be sensitive to the patient's response to all inquiry, and to respond to questions. In particular, it almost always helps to reassure the patient that items being inquired about are routine and that the student has not noticed something to make him suspicious.]*

DOC/PT: Besides the cortisone for your colitis, a lot more specifics now about major league treatments you might ever have had: blood transfusions (no), insulin (no), digitalis (no), or anti-coagulants (no). *[This is an additional way of screening for any major problems not yet mentioned.]*

DOC: Any visits to your doctor during the last year or so for anything we haven't covered?

PT: Well, I did have a bladder infection once and got some medicine for it.

DOC: What were your symptoms? *[The student is not taking her word for the diagnosis and, rightly, wants to know the symptoms, and will want to know any secondary data.]*

PT: One morning when I woke up I had to go all the time—and it burned, and I'd have to go all of a sudden, but I felt okay.

DOC: When was this?

PT: Last July, just before the fourth.

DOC: How long did it last?

PT: Oh, with the medicine it was gone in about 2 days, but I took the medicine for a week.

DOC: Did the pain, the burning, move anyplace like up into the bladder or back?

PT: No.

DOC: How many times a day would you go?

PT: Oh, that first day it must have been every hour.

DOC: Anything help it?

PT: Just the medications.

DOC/PT: Any of these symptoms go with it? fever (no), chills (no), blood in the urine (no), back pain (no), pass anything in the urine (no), getting up at night (a couple times when it started), unable to pass urine (no), or unable to control your bladder (no). *[Again, these are addressed individually.]*

DOC: Any tests done, like looking up in your bladder or cultures of the urine?

PT: No, she just gave me some medicine, a sulfa drug of some kind.

DOC: Ever had this before?

PT: Nope, it didn't amount to much. *[The student has a good profile of pertinent symptoms from the urinary system, knows the attendant secondary data, and has established the chronology of what sounds like an uncomplicated lower urinary tract infection. This is a simple and straight-forward problem, but the interviewer would evaluate each significant (to present health) PMH problem in a similar fashion.]*

DOC: Any other problems you've seen your doctor or anyone else for?

PT: No.

DOC: If there's nothing else, I'd like to shift and find out about medications and some other things. *[A good open-ended start into this new area. Because of space constraints, we'll simply summarize the student's findings. Except for the birth control pills and aspirin (detailed dosages and other data obtained) with the headaches, she's taking no medications or other treatments from either prescribed or other sources. The history of prednisone is reviewed. She has no allergic diseases and there is no history of adverse reactions to any drugs or other substances. Her menstrual and obstetric history are recounted in the write-up in Appendix B.]*

Social History (Step 10)

The social history (SH), also called the psychosocial history or the patient profile, provides two types of data: (1) the details, if any, of current personal or psychological problems not obtained in the HPI/OCAP, and (2) routine personal data about noncurrent issues [9,10].

The SH completes, if necessary, the personal profile begun during the patient-centered process, guided by the "current personal situation" category. Although often much of the information in the social history outline, presented below, has been obtained, it provides guidelines for additional specific details that sometimes must be addressed, as shown in the following vignette.

Social History (Step 10)*
1. Current personal situation
   a. Demographic: age, sex, race, current work and living situation
   b. Impact (meaning) of illness on self and others
   c. Beliefs/explanations about illness
   d. Relationships and support system
   e. Practical issues
   f. Stress
   g. Financial situation

2. Other personal factors
   a. Early developmental outline: birth and early development, early family setting and other caretakers, relationship with parents and siblings, others' relationships in family, early schooling and progress, places of residence, major losses and other adverse events, medical-surgical problems, happy events, later education and progress, social life and relationships, dating, adolescence, military or other service, getting away from home
   b. Marriage/other relationships and outcome: significant relationships (origin, course, outcome), children
   c. Work history and outcome: jobs and duration, satisfaction, toxic or other dangerous exposure (fumes, radiation, noise, dusts, chemicals)
   d. Recreational history
   e. Retirement
   f. Aging
   g. Life satisfaction
   h. Cultural/ethnic background

---

*Adapted from Morgan WL, Engel GL. *The Clinical Approach to the Patient*. Philadelphia: Saunders, 1969; and Billings AJ, Stoeckle JD. *The Clinical Encounter: A Guide to the Medical Interview and Case Presentation*. Chicago: Year Book, 1989.

As in the HI and PMH, the student obtains the SH by screening open-ended questions (requests) followed by closed-ended questions for details. Also like the HI and PMH, while it is not the intent to return to the patient-centered process, the interviewer does so if significant issues or emotions develop, or if a previously reticent patient begins to open up. It is not uncommon to go back and forth between patient-centered and doctor-centered processes many times.

Because the "other personal factors" category is potentially very extensive, the experienced clinician focuses on the "current personal situation" data so that the SH is obtained in a timely way, often only completing the entire SH over many visits. The bottom line is to better understand the patient and fill in any necessary gaps. Beginning clinical level students, however, obtain answers to all items. This is essential for learning the questions and understanding the many dimensions of human beings.

Continuation of Vignette of Mrs. Jones

DOC: We need to shift gears again and get some more details about your personal situation. *[A nice transition]*

PT: Seems like I've told you everything.

DOC: Well, I need to get a few more details. First, though, how are you doing with all this questioning? *[Always attending primarily to the patient's needs, the student takes time to inquire about the process of the interview itself.]*

PT: No problem. I like how thorough you are: *[She is doing well and makes a positive comment about the interviewer, indicating that a good relationship exists.]*

DOC: Thanks. Sometimes it feels like pressure to get so many questions. I appreciate your patience. Now, I need to get some more information. How old are you? *[The student is beginning to get some basic demographic data. Age is sometimes asked much earlier for basic orientation.]*

PT: Thirty-eight and just had a birthday.

DOC: And your family has been here for how long? *[The student is not clear how long she has actually been in the city.]*

PT: About 4 months.

DOC: I think I know the answer to this but I'll ask anyway. How have these headaches affected you and your family's lives? *[Open-ended inquiry about impact of the headaches. Although the patient has not raised the issue of impact, the student can introduce it in the SH. The doctor-centered process allows the interviewer to take the lead to obtain necessary details about personal data.]*

PT: It's been very disruptive. We were always quite happy and enjoyed things together. I told you about our sex life, and now the kids seem to get on my nerves all the time, too. Things need to get settled down. The job, not just the headaches. I'm not sure I'd stay in this job if things don't change.

DOC: It's been a difficult time. I do think we can help with the headaches, but I don't know about your boss. *[Interspersing a patient-centered intervention, here with naming and supporting statements, continues to be important.]*

PT: He's supposed to retire in 6 months. If the headache comes around, I can make it that long.

DOC: I know you think the headaches are from your boss, but any other ideas why you might be getting them? *[The student is leading and shifting away from her boss and probing for any other beliefs about why she is ill.]*

PT: Only punishment! I was raised with that always there. *[Depending on the amount of time available, one could return to the patient-centered process and explore this, allowing Mrs. Jones' ideas to lead. On the other hand, it is not current and she is exhibiting no distress so that it also can comfortably be left until another time.]*

DOC: Punishment? *[The student could not resist such a loaded clue and follows up open-endedly by echoing.]*

PT: Well, in our school — grade school mostly — we were told God would punish us when we were bad.

DOC: Say more. *[An open-ended request, now back in the patient-centered process with Mrs. Jones leading the conversation.]*

PT: You'd go to hell or die or get injured or something like that (tensely and seriously).

DOC: Say more about the school. *[Another open-ended request]*

PT: It was awful. They hit our hands with rulers all the time. If you didn't now the Bible lesson for the day — an hour each day no less! — you got hit and kept after school. I'd forgotten that, kind of.

DOC: What's the feeling that went with that? *[Emotion-seeking]*

PT: Guilt, I think — feeling bad, like I was bad or something. *[Mrs. Jones seems to be describing shame rather than guilt as we begin to learn yet another dimension of her story and consider, perhaps, how this fits the rest of the picture.]*

DOC: Where'd your mother fit into this? *[This is patient-centered because the interviewer already has heard about Mrs. Jones' mother and their conflict; the latter makes it relevant. The student wonders (hypothesizes) about the mother's role; for example, was she punitive herself, what did she think of the school practices, what did she do about them? Notice that the student did not use an emotion-handling response here; they are not used with every expression of emotion and sometimes are better deferred so that one can first deepen the story.]*

PT: Well, she didn't like it much either but it was the only school there.

DOC: It sounded earlier like your mother was kind of punitive. *[This is an open-ended summary of what the student already had heard during the initial patient-centered process. As long* *as it is germane, as it is here, it is appropriate to reintroduce such material. It is this type of "pushing" that we must do to deepen the story, always of course attending to the patient's response and readiness to follow her/his story to deeper levels.]*

PT: Yeah, I guess you could say that. Now that I think of it, I guess she was.

DOC: That wasn't an easy time growing up. *[Instead of pursuing the story still deeper, the student changes to emotion-handling with a respecting statement that acknowledges Mrs. Jones' plight as a youngster. This understanding and the previous understanding are remarkable accomplishments for a beginning clinical level student—to have effectively probed so deeply during the first interview. As one's skills with the interview improve and as knowledge of basic human dynamics increases, students will be able to take such a story even more deeply when the need arises.]*

PT: It sure wasn't.

DOC: Well, you seemed to come out of it okay. *[Another respecting statement, this time praising her for how well she seems to have done in spite of these problems.]*

PT: Thanks.

DOC: If it's okay to change, I'd like to ask you something else (she nods approval). You mentioned your husband earlier. Anybody else around that you can talk with? *[This recent dialogue shows how one returns to the patient-centered process. Mrs. Jones, although not distressed, had raised some important information that the student wanted to learn more about and could do so only by such a brief shift out of the doctor-centered process. The student has learned some important data, determined that Mrs. Jones is not upset, and has her approval to change the subject. He now closed-endedly begins to explore Mrs. Jones' support network.]*

PT: There's another new person there with the same problem and we commiserate all the time. He's taking over in another area but has the same boss. We get along great and seem to help each other. And, a couple other guys there know what's going on and have been very helpful—and had some good advice: Stay away from him. *[As with the rest of this dialogue, nothing urgent is arising so the student, recalling the need to be timely, simply obtains the information and doesn't pursue these issues in any depth.]*

DOC: Is it possible to avoid him? *[A closed-ended question addressing a very practical personal issue that has therapeutic implications, once again showing how inextricable is the link of disease and the personal dimension.]*

PT: Actually, it is. I have to do a lot of traveling and can schedule it around him and things are much better then. I figured it out and I can miss him for at least half the time in the next 6 months! *[If it weren't possible to avoid him and treat the headaches, the student and Mrs. Jones would have a bigger problem on their hands. In that event, this could be further addressed now or, more likely, at a subsequent visit that might be set up specifically for developing a strategy.]*

DOC: You've sure had a lot of stress. Are financial issues a problem, you know like medical insurance or anything? *[Changing the subject to another important potential problem that must be raised by closed-ended means.]*

PT: No! That was one of the benefits here. They cover everything with their insurance plan. I only pay a few dollars for everything, even medicines.

DOC: Let me shift a little and ask about some of your childhood. *[The student has now explored salient SH areas for current personal situation issues and is beginning to obtain some of the more routine information not relating to current personal issues. Mrs. Jones' situation is admittedly very straightforward and she is a bright, resourceful patient. The circumstances and details, however, don't always fall together so easily and this inquiry can take much longer. Because of space constraints, we will not recount the remainder of the SH but, rather, indicate that the student inquired about each remaining item in the SH outline that had not already been covered. This information can be found in the written report of Mrs. Jones in Appendix B.]*

Family History (Step 11)

The family history (FH) is another rich source for completing the personal database when necessary [9,10]. The student most wants to know who is who, and who is available to the patient and in what way. In general, the FH includes information for at least two generations preceding the patient, as well as for any subsequent generations, and includes parents, siblings, and children for each generation. Although not significant for familial or heritable disorders, this includes spouses, adoptees, and other significant members of the family outside the bloodline.

Family History (step 11)*
1. General inquiry
2. Inquire about specific diseases or problems: tuberculosis, diabetes, cancer, heart disease, bleeding problems, kidney failure or dialysis, alcoholism, tobacco use, weight problems, asthma, and mental illness (depression, suicide, schizophrenia, multiple somatic complaints)
3. Develop a genogram
   a. Two generations preceding the patient and all subsequently; includes parents, siblings, children, and significant members outside the bloodline for each generation
   b. Age, sex, mental and physical health, and current status are noted for each; note age at death and cause
   c. Note interactions among family members for psychological and physical/disease problems
      (1) Psychological
         (a) Dominant members and style (e.g., love, anger, alcoholism)
         (b) Major interaction patterns (e.g., competition, abuse, open, distant, caring, manipulation, codependent)
         (c) family gestalt (e.g., happy, successful, losers)
      (2) Physical/disease
         (a) Patterns of disease (e.g., dominant, recessive, sex-linked, no pattern)
         (b) Patterns of physical symptoms without disease (e.g., bowel trouble, uncoordinated, flighty)
         (c) Inquire about others with similar symptoms (e.g., infection, toxicity, anxiety)

---

*Adapted from Morgan WL, Engel GL. *The Clinical Approach to the Patient*. Philadelphia: Saunders, 1969; Billings AJ, Stoeckle JD. *The Clinical Encounter: A Guide to the Medical Interview and Case Presentation*. Chicago: Year Book, 1989; and Mullins HC, Christie-Seely J. Collecting and Recording Family Data—The Genogram. In Christie-Seely J (ed.), *Working with the Family in Primary Care: A Systems Approach to Health and Illness*. New York: Praeger, 1984. Pp. 179–191.

Once again, the interviewer uses open-to-closed coning inquiry to obtain the material noted in the outline. After a screening open-ended question ("Tell me about any illnesses or other problems running in your family"), specific diseases are mentioned: tuberculosis, diabetes, cancer, heart disease, bleeding problems, kidney failure or dialysis, alcoholism, tobacco use, weight problems, asthma, and mental illness (depression, schizophrenia, multiple somatic complaints, suicide, violence).

The student constructs a genogram to organize these data [15]. As noted in Mrs. Jones' genogram in Appendix B, this graphic form depicts myriad features in the family. Ages, gender, state of mental and physical health, and current status are obtained for each; when deceased, the age and cause of death are noted. Depending on time, data can profitably be extended to include education, work, psychological style, and a host of other features for each member.

The interviewer also learns about dominant and nondominant family members, and their specific styles; for example, controlling, passive, caring. In addition to individual psychological profiles, the interactions among family members (e.g., direct, indirect, conflicted, close) are equally important. One also ascertains the gestalt of the family and its unique persona; for example, the patient came from a successful family or a fighting family.

The classic use of the FH has been to obtain data about organic diseases by providing information about contagious (pinworm, varicella), toxic (carbon monoxide, lead), familial (breast cancer, coronary artery disease), and heritable (hemophilia, sickle cell anemia) diseases. In screening for these, the student asks if anyone in the family has similar physical problems to the patient's, or if anyone at home has been ill lately with similar complaints.

Many patients, however, report illnesses in the family that do not refer to the same disorder ("my father had a heart attack and I've got a murmur" likely refers to different problems), or even to any disease at all ("we all have bowel trouble"). Finally, especially following a relative's death, the patient may worry that they are at increased risk because of familial connections; for example, a healthy 21-year-old presents with chest pain and worries about having a heart attack 10 days after her grandfather died suddenly of a myocardial infarction. Most of these symptoms relate to the patient's understandable concern. While not the intent of the FH, students prepare to become supportive and address emotional material if it arises; for example, if, in discussing the dates of death of his parents, the patient becomes sad and tearful. As before, returning to the patient-centered process is essential.

With the large amount of potential data, the FH focuses on family data relevant to current problems. Students, however, again are urged to obtain all FH data in order to learn the categories themselves and the richness and variablity of the FH in different people. Busy clinicians often must acquire these data over many visits.

Continuation of Vignette with Mrs. Jones

DOC: Well, that's a lot of information. You've sure had a lot going on (referring to the SH). We've still got a little more information to gather and need to switch now to your family. *[The student continues to weave a patient-centered, respectful atmosphere into his comments to Mrs. Jones, and is making yet another transition, now into the FH.]*

PT: That's fine.

DOC: Are there any medical problems in your family, you know illnesses or any problems? *[Focused, open-ended beginning]*

PT: Nothing really. You made me think earlier about that one aunt who had some kind of headaches.

DOC: Even besides headaches, is there anything running in the family? *[The student makes sure Mrs. Jones knows that any familial problem is being inquired about.]*

PT: Well, my grandmother had diabetes; is that what you mean?

DOC/PT: Yeah, that's it. Let me give you some things and tell me if anyone in the family has it when I mention it: tuberculosis (no), kidney failure (no), bleeding problems (no), heart attacks (no), alcoholism (no), tobacco use (no), or mental problems (no). *[This helps the patient understand what is being requested and the student screens for a number of diseases of possible familial origin, each asked individually.]*

DOC: I need now to get some information on your immediate family, and then we'll go to your parents' and grandparents' families. Can you start by giving me the ages of your kids and your husband? *[The student begins a list of each family member of this and the preceding two generations, which will include ages, sex, mental and physical health, and their current status. We will not recount the interview here because of space constraints but Mrs. Jones' genogram is presented in Appendix B. Note the interactions among many members.]*

DOC: Well, we're just about done. Before we go on, though, how are you doing?

PT: A little weary but I'm fine.

DOC: You've been very helpful. Anything I can do for you before we go on? *[Once again, the student returns to the patient-centered process and attends to the patient's needs.]*

System Review (Review of Systems) (Step 12)

The review of systems (ROS) is less important than other parts of the history [16]; we already have discussed the system review in another context (a resource that lists most symptoms) in Chapter 4, where a detailed list occurs. Indeed, by this point, the interviewer ordinarily knows everything of significance. The ROS is not used for obtaining pertinent HPI/OCAP, HI, or PMH data and, rather, serves only as a final screening [9,10,16]. Indeed, recall that OCAP data often occur after repeated inquiries of "What else?" during agenda-setting (step 2)—which means that little if any new, important, or current data should arise here. Nonetheless, relevant data are sometimes acquired [17]; the student then fits them into the HPI/OCAP, HI, or PMH during the write-up or presentation.

The ROS concerns primary and secondary data from systems not yet considered. The interviewer returns to the system review and inquires about unaddressed symptoms and any secondary data, including specific diseases (e.g., psoriasis, cataracts).

The student often learns about many minor problems; for example, when screening for nasal symptoms, the patient wants to relate each cold and upper respiratory illness they have had over the last 20 years. Rather than obtaining details, the student wants to know only if the problem has been out of the ordinary, has caused any disability, represents a significant change, or has not completely cleared. Refocusing the patient helps, with comments such as "I don't need all the details, but I do want to know if there have been any other major problems." As before, recalling the need to be timely and not to overtax the patient, unnecessary data are not collected. In like fashion, one does not probe for or encourage symptoms. Most frustrating is the patient who answers positively to most questions, exhibiting a "positive system review." If this persists following clarification, it suggests still unrecognized diseases or a psychological disorder known as somatization in which patients present with multiple physical complaints that have no disease explanation.

The ROS proceeds almost entirely by rapidly paced, brief closed-ended questioning after an initial, orienting question such as "I need to ask you now about any other important or current problems or symptoms you might have had, so we don't miss something." For example, if the gastrointestinal system had not yet been addressed, the interviewer might begin open-endedly with "Any trouble with your digestion or bowels?" and then inquire "Have you ever had trouble with your appetite?" (No); "Weight loss?" (No); "Weight gain?" (No); "Difficulty swallowing?" (No); "Nausea?" (No); and so on until all of this system has been explored. Questions, of course, are asked and answered individually. When the more advanced clinical student has memorized all symptoms on the system review list, and is no longer confused by doing two things at once, she is urged to intersperse ROS material when performing the physical examination—as a time-saving device. For example, while one examines the nose, questions about nasal symptoms are asked; while examining the eyes, questions about the eyes are asked; and so on. One always remains attentive to the patient's responses and needs, and tells him that questions are "routine" and that the student has not noticed something to make her suspicious.

When the ROS is concluded, the student summarizes briefly, asks if the patient has anything else, and usually indicates that the physical examination will follow. A patient-centered atmosphere of courtesy, respect, and support continues throughout.

Final Vignette of Mrs. Jones

DOC: I need to ask you now about some symptoms we haven't yet talked about, you know, to be sure we haven't missed something so far. *[An effective open-ended introduction to the ROS.]*

PT: Fine, but I don't think there's much more.

DOC: We haven't talked yet about any skin problems; any problems there? *[An open-ended introduction to the integument system.]*

PT: I thought I had some infection in my elbow once in 1980, but it turned out I'd used too strong a soap. It's cleared long ago.

DOC/PT: Any problems since (no) or other skin problems like sores (no), itching (no), rashes (no), changes in moles (no), abnormal hair growth (no), or nail problems (no)? *[The student is getting an idea of how significant this is to Mrs. Jones' current* *health and then completes the ROS for the integument-related system.]*

DOC: *[The student would now proceed to other systems not yet addressed and inquire about all possible symptoms in each, as outlined on pp. 58–63 of Chapter 4; for example, hemopoietic, endocrine, breasts, genital. At its conclusion, he would conclude the interview as noted next.]*

DOC: Well, you've told me a lot about the problems with headaches and your boss, and about the colitis. I think I have a very good picture of what's going on. Is there anything else you'd like to add? *[A brief summary, understanding, support for her performance, and a patient-centered invitation for any final words.]*

PT: No, I don't think so.

DOC: In that case, I'll step out now so you can get undressed and I'll be back in a few minutes for the physical examination. If you'd like to use the bathroom or get a drink of water, please do. *[Further material about the transition to the physical examination in a respecting, patient-centered way.]*

Summary

In the doctor-centered HPI/OCAP, the interviewer converts complaints to one of the symptoms in the system review and then refines them with the seven descriptors. He then orders primary and secondary data into chronological sequence, progressively learning to test disease hypotheses as he proceeds. Health issues (HI) inquiry concerns ethical-social-spiritual issues, functional status, health-promoting and health-maintenance activities, and various health hazards. The PMH mainly recounts important but not current problems. The SH and FH complete the personal and, to a lesser extent, the primary and secondary database. The ROS screens for still undetected primary and secondary data.

By the repeated coning-down process of brief open-ended screening followed by closed-ended acquisition of necessary details, the interviewer better understands previous personal and symptom data from the patient-centered process and, in addition, acquires other essential parts of the database to complete the interview. Although not now as prominent, the student returns to a patient-centered process frequently by making supportive comments and inquiring how the patient is doing, and the interviewer returns to more extensive patient-centered, open-ended inquiry when the patient becomes emotional or presents important, new personal data.

References

1. Elstein AS. Psychological Research on Diagnostic Reasoning. In Lipkin M, Putnam SM, Lazare A, (eds.), *The Medical Interview*. New York: Springer-Verlag, 1995. Pp. 504–510.
2. Barrows HS, Pickell GC. *Developing Clinical Problem-Solving Skills — A Guide to More Effective Diagnosis and Treatment*. New York: Norton Medical Books, 1991.
3. Elstein AS, et al. Methods and theory in the study of medical inquiry. *J Med Educ* 47:85–92, 1972.
4. Sackett DL, Haynes RB, Tugwell P. *Clinical Epidemiology: A Basic Science for Clinical Medicine*. Boston: Little, Brown, 1985.
5. Griner PF, Panzer RJ, Greenland P. *Clinical Diagnosis and the Laboratory: Logical Strategies for Common Medical Problems*. Chicago: Year Book, 1986.
6. Sox HC. *Common Diagnostic Tests: Use and Interpretation*. Philadelphia: American College of Physicians, 1987.
7. Platt FW. *Conversation Repair*. Boston: Little, Brown, 1995.
8. Kuhn CC. A spiritual inventory of the medically ill patient. *Psychiatr Med* 6:87–100, 1988.
9. Morgan WL, Engel GL. *The Clinical Approach to the Patient*. Philadelphia: Saunders, 1969.
10. Billings AJ, Stoeckle JD. *The Clinical Encounter — A Guide to the Medical Interview and Case Presentation*. Chicago: Year Book, 1989.
11. Clark W. Effective Interviewing and Intervention for Alcohol Problems. In Lipkin M, Putnam SM, Lazare A (eds.). *The Medical Interview*. New York: Springer-Verlag, 1995. Pp. 284–293.
12. Williams S. The Sexual History. In Lipkin M, Putnam SM, Lazare A (eds.). *The Medical Interview*. New York: Springer-Verlag, 1995. Pp. 235–246.
13. Medical Economics. Physicians' Desk Reference (48th ed.). Montvale, NJ: Medical Economics Data Production Company, 1994.
14. Eisenberg DM, et al. Unconventional medicine in the United States: prevalence, costs, and patterns of use. *N Engl J Med* 328:246–252, 1993.
15. Mullins HC, Christie-Seely J. Collecting and Recording Family Data: The Genogram. In Christie-Seely J (ed.), *Working with the Family in Primary Care: A Systems Approach to Health and Illness*. New York: Praeger, 1984. Pp. 179–191.
16. Hoffbrand BI. Away with the system review: a plea for parsimony. *Br Med J* 298:817–818, 1989.
17. Mitchell TL, et al. Yield of the screening review of systems: A study on a general medicine service. *J Gen Intern Med* 7:393–397, 1992.

6

Practical Issues

The student must learn to fine-tune the interview and adapt it to many clinical situations, and does so primarily during steps 1 through 5 (setting the stage, agenda-setting, nonfocused interviewing, focused interviewing, and transition). This chapter focuses only on the interviewing process and does not consider details of the specific clinical situations. Readers are referred to clinical texts and to interviewing resource texts [1] to obtain the clinical details that must be incorporated into the interviewing process discussed here.

Balancing Patient-Centered and Doctor-Centered Processes

Even though the student knows how much time she can spend with the patient, there is no fixed rule on how to distribute the time between the patient-centered and doctor-centered processes. Based on the patient's needs, the interviewer determines the initial balance during steps 1 through 5. We might average 10 percent of our time in the initial patient-centered process for most patients, but this allocation of time can vary from 2 percent (e.g., a patient who needs a medication refill and has no personal issues) to more than 50 percent (e.g., a patient with severe marital problems), depending on the severity and urgency of the patient's personal issues. Of course, it also may be necessary to return again and again to a patient-centered approach even late in the interview.

During the patient-centered process, the interviewer's main block of controllable time lies in step 4, focused interviewing. Steps 1 through 3 and step 5 usually take little time and are similar from patient to patient. Consider the following examples.

New Patient Without Urgent
or Complex Personal Problems

First consider a prototypical new patient, like Mrs. Jones, who comes to the doctor without urgent (where immediate action is required) or complex personal problems. Physical symptom complaints often predominate and the interviewer usually devotes about 10 percent of time to the initial patient-centered process of the interview. This will be the student's experience with most new patients in a medical setting, whether outpatient or inpatient. Such patients, like Mrs. Jones, have definite personal issues but they are not urgent or overwhelming; for example, a patient with known cancer is admitted to the hospital for chemotherapy but is more worried about his wife being alone and having the flu; an outpatient presents with a weight loss of 5 pounts and is somewhat concerned about possible cancer and wants "to be sure."

New Patient with Urgent or Complex Personal Problems

There are, however, new in- or outpatients with more urgent and complex personal problems; for example, acute marital discord led to sleeplessness, depression, headaches, and diarrhea for this outpatient who requested a "check-up"; or a recent unexpected business setback immediately preceded the admission to the hospital of this now very angry man with chest pain; or a patient admitted for pneumonia who is overwhelmed and crying after being informed of an AIDS diagnosis. In these instances, the student gives more time to personal issues by increasing time in step 4 and, very likely, the interviewer also will spend time during the doctor-centered process (steps 6 and 7) to better understand details of what could be a serious psychological problem (see p. 92 of Chap. 5). If, for example, Mrs. Jones had shown evidence of depression or inability to function at work, the patient-centered process would have taken considerably longer.

Follow-Up Patient Without Urgent
or Complex Personal Problems

Just as with new patients, most follow-up patients do not have urgent or complex personal problems but they differ in having much less time with the student. Consider a follow-up visit, either inpatient or outpatient, for predominantly physical complaints. The student quickly proceeds through steps 1–4 and ascertains there are few pressing personal issues for this brief visit. She will then shorten step 4 and make a transition (step 5) into the doctor-centered process (steps 6 and 7) where the just-determined agenda about the patient's physical symptoms is addressed; for example, any worsening or new symptoms after treating the patient's Strep throat 1 week ago; or any change from the preceding day in this inpatient's chest pain. In both instances, the student listens for new personal contextual material (wants to get back to work, wants to go home) and responds, but most personal data already will be known and the patient's symptoms will be the primary focus. The personal issues of follow-up patients often concern treatment and disposition. Because the database is more complete, we can more easily investigate treatment issues during the patient-centered process than we can with new patients.

Vignette of Mr. Gomez

(Ward rounds on a patient with primarily physical symptoms on his second day of hospitalization, with no more than 15 minutes available at this time)

DOC: (Observes patient for comfort, helps with pillow, and sits down.) Anything new you'd like me to look at today before I do some of my things (pointing to stethoscope)? *[The student sets the stage by attending to the patient's comfort, gives her own agenda (stethoscope), and asks about the patient's agenda so that both steps 1 and 2 are addressed in no more than a few seconds.]*

PT: Nothing new.

DOC: How you doing? *[An open-ended question to start step 3]*

PT: The pain is better. Can I go home? *[The patient gives both symptom and personal data.]*

DOC: Go home?

PT: Ya, my job. Remember, we talked about it?

DOC: Sure, anything new?

PT: No, but they still need me and my wife's in a fix.

DOC: Well, I sure understand you're anxious about your job and that's sure a tough situation for your wife to be in, but there's a little more. Our (pointing to the patient and herself) biggest concern now is to be certain you are okay and don't have an appendicitis, and we aren't sure yet. *[Note that, in a brief visit, the student addresses the personal issue to start step 4, but does not reexplore what she already knows except to ascertain no change. The student also incorporates naming, understanding, and support into her response. The re-*

sponse was supportive both verbally and nonverbally, involving the patient by pointing and using the terms "our" and "we".]

PT: You still think tomorrow?

DOC: Well, if the blood count and x-ray turn out okay and the pain clears up, it's possible. But don't count on it yet. Our main need now is your health and getting you back to your job in good shape. Sounds really difficult for you, though. *[The student continues addressing personal issues in step 4 by staying focused on the question raised by the patient and again makes a supportive statement, about wanting most to help the patient, and a respecting statement.]*

PT: Yeah, thanks. *[The patient seems satisfied]*

DOC: Let me shift now and have you tell me more about the pain. *[This is step 5, the transition, and a beginning of step 6 of the doctor-centered process still using open-ended requests. Note that the student effectively conducted the patient-centered process in about 1 minute and now will address the patient's medical condition in steps 6 and 7.]*

PT: Well, the pain yesterday was more around the belly button but now it's down here on the right (right lower quadrant). It hurts to push on it but isn't bad otherwise.

DOC: Any bowel movement yet? . . . *[The student will spend the next several minutes determining symptom descriptors, if symptoms are changed from yesterday, and search out and define any new symptoms. She will then examine the patient, review the laboratory data, and make further plans. Steps 8–12 of the doctor-centered process will be unnecessary because the student obtained these data when the patient was admitted to the hospital the previous day. The student also will inform the patient that she will be back when the results of the lab tests and x-ray are available. Note again how closely the patient's personal issues revolve about the symptom.]*

Such a predominantly doctor-centered follow-up interaction also can concern personal data. When the student wants to address a specific issue that the patient has not raised, such as sexual habits or cigarette cessation, this also requires that most time be spent in the doctor-centered process.

Follow-Up Patient with Urgent or Complex Personal Problems

On the other hand, we may have a follow-up patient presenting urgent or complex personal issues, often but not always with few physical complaints. The interviewer quickly determines this during steps 1 through 4, and then takes more time in step 4 to better develop the personal issues, resulting in a predominantly patient-centered interview. Even with no physical complaint expressed by the patient, however, the student makes a transition to the doctor-centered process and briefly inquires about the patient's physical health; for example, "No more problems with the heartburn or constipation?" That is, one always integrates the personal and symptom data.

Vignette of Mrs. Wong

(An outpatient previously seen for other problems now presents with a predominantly personal problem in a 20-minute appointment slot.)

DOC: Hi, Mrs. Wong. Hadn't seen you for awhile. Is that comfortable sitting there? (she nods) Anything you need before we get started? *[step 1]*

PT: No, unless you can fix my son. He is getting a divorce. And that means the grandchildren will have to leave town. And then . . . *[The patient is introducing tension-laden personal material already.]*

DOC: That sounds pretty heavy. We're going to need to get back to this in a minute but before we get started, could you tell me if there was anything else you wanted to look at today, you know, other problems? *[The student determines that it is appropriate, as is usually the case, to briefly interrupt in order to get the agenda (step 2).]*

PT: Well, I came because of my back. It's a little worse and you did all those tests a year ago that were okay. I think it's the stress.

DOC: Anything else to look at today? *[The student is being certain that the entire agenda is elicited.]*

PT: No, that's enough!

DOC: So, tell me more about your son. Sounds like a tough time for you. *[When the patient has already begun with strongly felt personal data, it is appropriate to return directly to the material raised.]*

PT: Well, they've been married for nearly 15 years and everything always seemed okay. I think they thought so too. And now this. She's just furious at him.

DOC: (Silence) *[The student is in the nonfocusing step 3 and simply letting the patient lead.]*

PT: He's always been a bit of a ladies-man and, well, that's caused problems before too.

DOC: Sounds like a tough time for you. How're you doing with all this? *[Beginning to grasp the problem and recalling the need to be timely, the student introduces step 4 by changing the focus to her emotions. The details of the son's problem are less important now and can be developed later if necessary.]*

PT: (Starting to cry) I'm mad at him for being so stupid. And I can't stand having to be away from the little kids. She'll get them and they'll move back to her home. (more crying) *[This story would now be developed in much the same way Mrs. Jones' story was; that is, active open-ended, emotion-seeking, and emotion-handling skills are used over and over in a cyclic way. The student obtains more details and learns that Mrs. Wong is depressed, as she was once before following her husband's death. We will now pick it back up to show the transition to the doctor-centered process.]*

DOC: You've sure been through a lot and I'm glad you've told me about it. Do you feel okay to change gears now so I can ask a few more questions? *[The student is in step 5 and checking to see if the patient is finished talking about this difficult problem.]*

PT: Sure, and thanks again for listening. I feel better.

DOC: I wanted to ask about your sleep. How's that going?

PT: Not very good.

DOC: Do you have trouble getting to sleep? *[Because the student has learned that Mrs. Wong is depressed, she is starting to inquire about physical (vegetative) symptoms that often accompany depression. In addition to sleep disturbances, she will learn that Mrs. Wong has a poor appetite and no longer enjoys previously enjoyable activities (anhedonia), further supporting the diagnosis of depression, an urgent problem that will require treatment. The student then ascertains, continuing to use predominantly closed-ended inquiry, that Mrs. Wong is not suicidal. We now pick up the conversation where the student is addressing the back pain that brought the patient in.]*

DOC: Well, that's been a hard time for you. Could you now say more about the backache? *[One must address symptoms, however insignificant they may seem or however much the patient downplays them. Note again how closely the symptoms and personal problems often are related.]*

PT: It's the same place. And it never did go down the leg after that one time 4 years ago. I don't think it's anything . . . *[During the next few minutes the student reviews the symptom descriptors and then examines the patient. When she has dressed, the student will make recommendations about the depression and the back pain.]*

Of course we see a spectrum of patients between the urgent and less urgent personal categories, and there is no way to predict how many physical symptoms will be present in either category. What does one do in the difficult situation where both personal and symptom data are plentiful, urgent, and complex? Careful agenda-setting (step 2) will define what seems most important to both doctor and patient. Even so, some issues may have to be deferred to a later appointment.

How Common Interviewing Situations Are Addressed

Even after one plans how to distribute time between the initial patient-centered and doctor-centered processes, there are still patient styles and situations that influence interviewing and affect how time will be spent; for example, a loquacious patient may require more time, more interruptions, and less encouragement than a reticent one to give the same story. Let us now consider some variations on our theme. As before, most decisions are made during steps 1 through 5.

The Reticent Patient
The interviewer must get reticent patients talking, about anything, whatever it takes. Typically, the agenda (step 2) is limited and about symptoms, and there is little response on the patient's part to initial open-ended inquiry (step 3). The nonfocusing open-ended skills (silence, nonverbal encouragement, neutral utterances) may be ineffective and, in step 4, the interviewer relies on the focusing open-ended skills (echoing, requests, summary) and

emotion-seeking skills (direct, indirect). Among the latter skills, self-disclosure is particularly effective; for example, "I once had chest pain and was very concerned, how about you?" Even though the patient may express no emotion, the student directs emotion-handling skills toward what she does know about the patient; for example, "It sounds like some difficult problems you've had; you were right to come in so we could help out" (naming, praising, supporting). This often facilitates additional information about the story.

To get some conversation going, the interviewer can talk about a patient's symptoms using closed-ended questions in step 4; for example, "What brings you in?" "Where is the back pain?" "Does it go down your leg?". Once the symptoms begin, one elicits their immediate personal dimensions and the broader personal context will follow. One looks for any thread of personal data to facilitate; for example, if the family dog is mentioned, focus on it to get some personal conversation going.

Ordinarily, these patients will talk and satisfactory stories can be elicited, albeit briefer and less complete than with other patients. Symptom data are easier to obtain from the doctor-centered process because the interviewer has more control of the conversation. Sometimes these patients offer personal data during the doctor-centered process, seemingly warmed up by what has preceded; for example, while giving the family history (FH), the patient begins to talk about personal issues. The student of course then alters her style to be patient-centered and further develops these personal data.

Such patients often frustrate and disappoint students, who often lament they "didn't get much." Although less is learned, the patient still feels understood and a good doctor-patient relationship develops. Research shows that doctors may encourage reticence with repeated closed-ended inquiries which lead to briefer and briefer answers [2]. The interviewer thus needs to be certain she is not thwarting the patient's ability to tell her story.

The Overly Talkative Patient

With overly talkative patients the interviewer tries to establish a personal and emotional focus in a timely way, especially focusing too detailed or diffuse conversation. These patients may begin without the interviewer's saying anything. Developing the agenda (step 2) typically is difficult. Nevertheless, the interviewer develops a list of complaints, often by interrupting and refocusing frequently. An open-ended beginning question is seldom necessary because patients already are giving much data. Indeed, silence alone often suffices as patients talk on in step 3. After no more than 1 to 2 minutes with a new patient (sooner with follow-up patients), the interviewer gets involved actively, lest she become nonparticipatory in step 4.

Some patients need to recount every detail. That sort of verbal output interferes with our getting personal and emotional data. The student must interrupt and redirect, sometimes repeatedly. Other patients discuss issues that don't relate to themselves directly; for example, about other people or politics. Still others focus on remote past events with no apparent relevance to their present situation. In all instances the interviewer actively refocuses the patient (step 4) on himself in the here and now ("I understand your concern about Clinton's health policy, but how does it apply to you, you know, personally?") and, in particular, their emotional reactions, using the emotion-seeking skills ("Those are important details, but how'd that affect you, emotionally?"). Also, the NURS tetrad (see Chap. 2) is a means by which the student can achieve a modicum of control of the interview; for example, "That's been a long spell for you. I can sure understand how upsetting it might be. Thanks for giving me that background. Let's move on now to what happened yesterday." On the other hand, if patients are talking about themselves in the present and giving emotional data, the student stays with them and facilitates this focus. Once such a focus is established, the interviewer's difficulty is to complete step 4 in a timely way. A firm, clear transition statement effectively changes focus to the doctor-centered process; for example, after summarizing and using the NURS tetrad, "We need now to change so I can learn more about your constipation if that's okay."

Talkative patients produce plentiful personal data and the interviewer may easily obtain a long story. Because of time constraints, the student avoids a prolonged return to such personal data if the patient reintroduces them later in the doctor-centered process. The most important data usually will already have arisen. Nonetheless, if emotion is expressed, one must address it. Briefly listening and using emotion-handling skills usually will suffice.

These patients can seem "easy" to the student inclined to passivity and "irritating" to those who themselves like to take control. Awareness of one's personal characteristics will maximize effectiveness. In Chapter 7, further strategies for addressing one's personal responses and for managing these patients are presented.

The Patient Who Persists in Symptoms and Secondary Data During the Patient-Centered Process

We now focus on a difficult, albeit uncommon, problem. When, after developing a good personal description of symptoms during the patient-centered process, the patient persists in physical symptoms and secondary data, the interviewer's strategy must change.

To encourage expanding the information to the general personal contextual data, open-ended skills are sometimes not enough and the interviewer may have to actively direct the patient with emotion-seeking skills. The symptoms pointing to medical disease in these patients may be prominent and fearful. One first summarizes this information and then follows immediately with emotion-seeking skills. Direct and indirect emotion-seeking inquiry typically establishes a personal focus. Respectful interrupting often facilitates the transition as well. As with the reticent patient, the personal stories often are more truncated and less complex.

These patients can be frustrating because the interview is difficult and because they are hard to get to know personally.

Vignette of Mr. Swenson

PT: (The patient has given limited personal descriptions of the following in steps 3 and 4, but without expression of concern, emotion, or anything more personal: arm pain, headache, loose stools, and nausea from medication. The patient also tells us of a negative CT scan and Dr. Johnson's diagnosis of arteritis.) *[The student knows that he is going to have to work harder than usual to draw out the broader personal context of these symptoms.]*

DOC: (first summarizes the physical problems and immediately follows with:) Boy, you've sure had a lot of things going on. How does that make you feel, you know, personally? *[Student summarizes symptoms and secondary data but directs patient toward its personal context by a direct emotion-seeking question.]*

PT: I don't know. This pain keeps going right over here. And I've also been coughing. That started last . . . (student interrupts) *[Patient is staying with symptoms and not responding with anticipated general personal contextual information; student interrupts quickly to try again to establish a more personal focus, otherwise the symptom focus will continue.]*

DOC: What I'm asking about are other things, like what you think is going on. Why's all this happening? *[Indirect emotion-seeking* *probing patient's beliefs is tried instead of repeating the direct inquiry about feelings.]*

PT: Dr. Johnson says it's arteritis. It's a blood vessel disease . . . (student interrupts) *[Student continues to look for personal clues but none yet—will keep trying.]*

DOC: But why you, why'd you get it? *[Persists in probe for beliefs; most patients have some opinion about this, which will lead to personal data.]*

PT: I don't know. *[The patient isn't saying much; student needs to use other indirect inquiry or return to direct inquiry about feelings.]*

DOC: With so much going on, how's it affected your life? *[Usually more productive indirect emotion-seeking inquiry because it forces some personal data; the patient can hardly say he doesn't know.]*

PT: Not much. I retired and wasn't doing anything anyway, until all this stuff came. That pain is right in . . . (student interrupts) *[At last, some personal data; the interviewer will now actively focus on this.]*

DOC: Tell me more about that, retiring and not doing much. *[Combined open-ended summary and request; now that personal data have appeared, focusing open-ended skills will be used repeatedly to maintain the focus and develop the personal story, as already described. Earlier, rather than indirect inquiry about beliefs and personal impact, the student could also have used self-disclosure or asked about the impact of illness on others' lives; if the patient lapses back into symptom data, these would be used now.]*

When Necessary Personal Data Are Not Forthcoming During the Patient-Centered Process

So far, we have assumed that the personal data we obtained during the patient-centered process are the most important personal data. Indeed, that is almost always so but such data aren't always complete, especially around topics where patients are embarrassed or fear others will perceive them as abnormal; for example, sexual practices, substance use, suicidal intent, and abuse.

Proceeding through steps 1 to 5, the interviewer often first suspects an occult problem; for example, a story of severe depression raises the question of suicidal intent or a story of frequent fractures raises the question of alcoholism. Sometimes, however, awareness does not arise until later (e.g., a story of recurrent pneumonia and diarrhea raises the question of AIDS and thereby homosexual activity or drug abuse, or one observes unusual bruises during the physical exam leading to thoughts of physical abuse).

Doctor-centered inquiry allows us to obtain the necessary information, usually at the start of the doctor-centered process (steps 6 and 7) although sometimes later on (e.g., HI, PMH, SH). The interviewer begins with a focused open-ended question ("I want to focus now on your use of alcohol") and follows up with progressively more closed-ended inquiry until all significant information is obtained. The HI section of Chapter 5 (step 8) shows the key data that must be elicited about sexual activity and addictive behaviors using this approach.

The interviewer should perform this inquiry with sensitivity and respect. He tells patients how important these data are to help them medically and reassures them of confidentiality. Almost invariably, the patient has some strong feelings that we must elicit with emotion-seeking skills and address using emotion-handling skills.

I recommend using the doctor-centered approach in this way whenever pertinent personal data are not obtained during patient-centered interviewing. For example, if the patient does not seem to be following treatment recommendations, the interviewer might start the doctor-centered process (steps 6 and 7) open-endedly with a question such as, "Let's talk about how you're taking each of your medicines each day," and follow up with more narrowly focused inquiry until clarity is achieved (e.g., "Let's count how many pills you have left in the container to be sure you're taking them like I think you are"). Thus, doctor-centered inquiry that is predominantly closed-ended often is required to supplement the personal database.

Students usually find it difficult to address issues that the patient is avoiding and has strong feelings about. The student herself may feel fear, concern, abhorrence, caring, or voyeuristic curiosity. Only an interviewer who is personally aware can keep these responses from interfering with her patient interaction.

When More than One Person Is Present

Although the family interview [3] is beyond the scope of this text, there are other situations where the student faces more than one person for the interview. The interviewer might decide to consult a relative or friend of the patient hoping he can provide unique information (e.g., a parent reporting on his child, what happened while the patient was unconscious, information the patient has forgotten or denied). A properly conducted interview involving a relative or other third person provides information otherwise unavailable, including how the patient interacts in this relationship; e.g., domineeringly, passively, distantly, angrily, or lovingly. Many hours of interviewing would be needed to provide as much "hard data" about the patient's interactional style. Perhaps a student obtains a story of great independence and achievement only to see the patient behave in a very dependent way when his spouse arrives. Or a person who appeared very sensitive and considerate during the interview becomes hostile and sharp with a family member.

During step 1, the student must first learn who the third party is and then learn if both the patient and third party want the third party present. Next, the interviewer asks whether the third party has special information she would like to convey. If this seems pressing, the student hears it out. The patient interview then takes place as described. The interviewer tries to monitor how the third party is doing, how she interacts with the patient, and what effect she has on learning about the patient. One weighs whether more or less data are being obtained because of the third party's presence. Problems can arise if the third party interrupts or nonproductively lengthens the interaction. This possibility has led many interviewers to reflexively dismiss all third parties. If they are interfering, the interviewer can focus on them, obtain other data they might have, and then respectfully excuse and thank them. Ensuring privacy while discussing sensitive issues and during physical examination are other reasons for excusing some third parties. On the other hand, relatives and friends often remain quiet. The interviewer may involve them for points requiring clarification or at the end of a successful interview to see how they view the problem (e.g., a spouse may see the patient as at great risk for cancer while the patient denies this; or a spouse may have practical questions the patient didn't raise).

The pressure of a group, often with an acutely ill or dying patient, provides another complex interaction. If it is possible to conduct an interview with the patient, the earlier guidelines obtain. The less responsive the patient, the more important the relatives, and the more important to identify who knows the most about the patient. Once the interviewer has attended to the patient's needs, she might consider her obligation to the relatives. They also need to be heard and understood. One listens to their concerns and emotions, uses emotion-handling skills, answers questions, and helps find solutions.

Involving third parties may take little time and produce data that otherwise would not be available. Nevertheless, the additional time required, the need to incorporate data from new sources, and having to focus on the needs of third parties do increase the demand on the student. Understanding one's own feelings of frustration (e.g., loss of control, aggravating an already inefficient approach, strict time orientation) can help the interviewer avoid adverse, often reflexive responses such as impatience, dismissing third parties, or avoiding relatives.

We must briefly consider the interview mediated by an interpreter [4]. When the third party is an interpreter (translating a foreign language, sign language, or for a dysarthric patient), the interaction takes considerably longer. At the outset, it helps to learn how much the interpreter already knows about the patient, what his relationship is, how well he understands the patient, and vice versa. Many interpreters are family members or friends and confidentiality is an issue; here, one also explores their relationship. Professional interpreters independent of the patient are best, but seldom available. Nonprofessional translators should be advised of the requirements of their job, for example, "I'm going to speak to your mother and she to me. I need you to translate exactly what I say and exactly what she says back. I know you'll be tempted to add or subtract because of what you know already but, for now, I need a precise translation only. Can you do that for me?". If the situation arises, one asks the interpreter to identify remarks as his own. One conducts the interview using the interpreter as the mediator, but addresses the patient directly, making eye contact and keeping her involved and central. The student is more directive and avoids jargon, technical terms, and abstractions. The student also periodically checks with the interpreter on the patient's nonverbal reactions, their understanding, and for culturally sensitive issues. Even with such an effort, the student may find it difficult to establish the usual relationship. The experience can be frustrating for patient and doctor alike. Indeed, it is helpful to acknowledge this [5]; for example, "It may be harder for us to get to know each other, but I want you to know I'm going to work on it." It helps to have the history written out in advance, by the patient or a knowledgeable relative, so the interviewer can focus on the relationship and major problems. It may be best for the patient to find a doctor who speaks the same language, especially for complicated or long-term care [5].

Patients with Communication Problems

Developing a patient-centered focus requires special attention when communication problems exist. The patient's handicap and the measures required to address it can distract the student from a patient-centered approach. We try not to overlook special needs such as allowing a deaf patient to see the interviewer's lips clearly, omitting usual needs such as touching the patient, and overcompensating for perceived but nonexistent needs such as speaking loudly and simply to a blind patient.

The relationship requires special attention. Nonverbal means can be especially effective and include touching the patient, a well-timed smile or friendly gesture, and an accepting demeanor [6]. Because of their impairment, many have been relatively isolated and are leery, particularly of insincere interactions, so that genuinely felt expressions that lead to a slower developing relationship are most effective [6]. Some who have speech or hearing impairment may seem cognitively impaired to the unwary interviewer who oversimplifies ideas and speech, often presenting material as though to a child [6].

It helps to have the history written in advance. This allows a more relaxed atmosphere and more focus on the relationship and key events. The following section presents additional measures that can enhance data-gathering and the relationship, often focusing on setting the stage for a successful interview and attending to comfort.

Hearing-Impaired

Most common with older patients, hearing impairment can cause great difficulty [7]. If the patient has a hearing aid, encourage the patient to use it. Inquire specifically about what can be most helpful. Patients appreciate the invitation and attention to their special needs, with which they are expert and have much experience in how best to communicate. Determine if the patient lip-reads and, if so, ensure that he can see the interviewer's face adequately. Reducing background noise, pointing, and using gestures also helps. Because the patient has learned to read lips of normally speaking people, the student should not slow down, shout, or overarticulate her speech. The student should speak at a moderate rate and volume, pause at the end of sentences, use complete sentences, and inform patients of changes in topics being discussed. When necessary, repeat statements using different words and write out certain words or ideas.

Mute
Writing is essential if a translator is not available for a signing patient and the student is not versed in sign language. With planning and instructions, the time required can be shortened by having others available who can provide information and by having the patient or others record the history before the visit.

Blind
Blind people, while communicating verbally in normal ways, lack many cues that sighted people routinely and unconsciously experience. Blind patients use auditory compensatory mechanisms to understand mood, style, friendliness, and other features of the interviewer. Such nonvisual cues are not necessarily in accord with what others would perceive, and it is important to pay special attention to their perceptions [6]; for example, the interviewer might ask, "Things are going okay for me, but I wanted to check with you how I'm coming across and how our interaction is going."

As before, it is useful to inquire if the blind patient has special ways of proceeding, if he needs assistance from the interviewer, if he has any particular requests relating to his blindness, and not to offer unwanted help. This allows him to take the lead and know that the interviewer is available and open to his needs—and respects his self-sufficiency [6]. Orientation to furniture and doors, others in the room, and the interviewer's movement during the history and physical examination are helpful. The interviewer's speech quality, intensity, and pace should remain normal and not be "adjusted" for the blind patient.

Cognitively Impaired
Cognitive disturbances present a different problem. Even though patients perceive and speak, they do not process the information intellectually in a normal way. Therefore, data are less reliable and meaningful, especially when the cognitive loss is severe.

Cognitive dysfunction is a vast topic that will be dealt with during clinical rotations in medicine, pediatrics, surgery, psychiatry, and neurology. Such dysfunction is common, can be acute or chronic, and may have many causes; for example, congenital, head injury, dementia, brain tumor, alcohol withdrawal, drug abuse, meningitis, medications, anemia, uremia, sepsis, hypoxia, poisoning, postoperative state. In addition, psychiatric disorders of mood, altered thinking, and abnormal mental experiences can present with cognitive changes as part of their presentation; for example, schizophrenia, depression [8,9].

To this point, we assumed that the patient was a reliable authority for primary and secondary data. Cognitively impaired patients often vary considerably in reporting symptoms with each telling and the chronology is typically unreliable. Similarly, emotions and other personal issues often are quite variable and nonreproducible. All told, these data often are incomplete and cannot be relied upon. The student needs to obtain external corroboration. Nonetheless, while gathering these data from family and others, one must attend to the patient's needs and to the relationship.

The interviewer begins in the usual way. With severe cognitive dysfunction, one easily recognizes the problem during steps 1 and 2: Patients don't know where they are, that they are in a medical setting, or who is with them. They make little sense and their stories are grossly inconsistent. There may be additional psychiatric symptoms (e.g., hallucinations) if the cognitive changes are part of a psychiatric problem. Mildly affected patients who remain aware that they are losing their cognitive capacities often compensate by keeping detailed notes of events and appointments to assist their failing memory, and carefully guard against showing evidence of cognitive dysfunction. Nevertheless, such loss of thinking capacity can be suspected during steps 1 through 5 by vagaries, inconsistencies, an undue focus on familiar areas, and deft circumventing of areas where memory has failed. The patient may use humor to mask confusion and failing memory. Unlike the more severe forms, we usually need systematic mental status evaluation to be certain. Once these problems are suspected, the interviewer shifts to the doctor-centered process (steps 6 and 7) and conducts systematic testing.

The content of a formal Mental Status Evaluation (MSE) is outlined below. Where inquiry is needed, rather than observation, it is conducted in the usual doctor-centered way, beginning with a general open-ended statement in relevant categories and pinning down details using closed-ended inquiry; for example, "Tell me about your memory (no problems). Good, I need to ask you some specific questions so we can get the details"; the interviewer then asks specific questions about important dates, and well-known facts ("Who is the President?"). Full MSE requires knowledge of the

Mental Status Evaluation*

1. Appearance: age, physical stigmata, dress, depression, general health, cleanliness, neatness
2. Attitude: cooperative, angry, guarded, suspicious, attentive, seductive, playful, obsequious
3. Activity: increased (hyperactivity, agitation), decreased, catatonic, abnormal movements (tics, tremors), visual-motor integrity
4. Mood (sustained objective emotional feeling): sad, happy, anxious, angry, depressed, detached, irritable
5. Affect (transitory, immediate emotional expression): full, flat, blunted, inappropriate, anhedonic, labile
6. Speech: normal, slowed, reduced, increased, pressured, mute, dysarthria, punning, rhyming
7. Language: bizarre, distracting, colorful, "word salad," circumstantial, tangential, loosening of associations, neologisms
8. Thought content: logical, incoherent, derailment, poverty of content, obsessive, delusional, paranoid
9. Perceptions: illusions, hallucinations (visual, auditory, olfactory, tactile), depersonalization, derealization
10. Judgment and insight: realistic, unrealistic, "la belle indifference"
11. Neuropsychiatric evaluation
    a. Level of consciousness: comatose, stuporous, drowsy, alert, hyperalert
    b. Attention and concentration: repeating digits, "serial 7s," spelling backwards, immediate memory
    c. Language function: fluency, comprehension, naming, repetition, reading, writing
    d. Memory: recent (orientation to time, place, and person; recall three unrelated objects); remote (past events); amnesia (retrograde, anterograde)
    e. Other higher functions: abstraction (proverbs), calculation, intelligence

*Adapted from Leon RL, Bowden, CL, Faber RA. The psychiatric interview, history, and mental status examination. In Kaplan HI, Sadock BJ (eds.). *Comprehensive Textbook of Psychiatry* (5th ed). v. 1. Baltimore: Williams & Wilkins, 1989. Pp. 449–462; and Andreason NC, Black DW. *Introductory Textbook of Psychiatry*. Washington, DC: American Psychiatric Press, Inc., 1991. Pp. 37–40.

various psychiatric, neurological, and medical conditions that cause abnormalities of mental status. Outlined in greater detail in standard clinical textbooks [8–11], the student makes observations or inquiry in the following areas, summarized in the outline.

Appearance

The student observes the gestalt or overall appearance of the patient: whether they appear older or younger than their age, the presence of unique physical attributes (prosthetic leg), their grooming and neatness, if they appear depressed or anxious, and their apparent state of health (ill appearing).

Attitude

The interviewer observes the patient's attitudes, both exhibited and expressed, during the interview, particularly for cooperativeness. Other attitudes include angry, guarded, suspicious, attentive, seductive, playful, and obsequious.

Activity

The student notes the patient's motor activity: increased (hyperactivity, agitation), decreased, catatonic, and abnormal movements (tics, tremors). One also asks the patient to draw a simple figure, such as a clock set at a specific time or a square inside a circle, to assess visual-motor integrity.

Mood

The student determines, primarily by inquiry, the patient's sustained, day-in and day-out, emotional feeling; for example, sad, happy, anxious, angry, depressed, detached, irritable.

Affect

Primarily by observation, the interviewer notes how the patient expresses his immediate emotional state. Is the patient fully and appropriately responsive to stimuli and circumstances? Or are his responses flat or blunted (dulled emotional responsivity), inappropriate (laughing when most would be serious), anhedonic (no enjoyment of anything), or labile? To combine mood and affect, one might say, "The patient's mood was depressed and the affect blunted."

Speech

Students observe for the following speech characteristics: normal, slowed, reduced, increased, pressured, mute, dysarthria, punning, rhyming.

Language

Interviewers observe the patient's use of language for the following characteristics: bizarre, distracting, colorful, word salad (incoherent mix of words and phrases seen in psychotic states), circumstantial, tangential, loosening of associations (connections that are difficult to follow), and neologisms (coining new words).

Thought Content

The student will determine the presence or absence, via the patient's speech and language, of the following characteristics of the patient's thought content: logical, incoherent, derailment, poverty of content, obsessive, delusional, paranoid. The student also notes the content of the thought, describing any delusions in detail. When thought is not logical and goal-oriented, serious problems exist.

Perceptions

The interviewer asks about abnormal perceptions, typically hallucinations that may be visual, auditory, olfactory, or tactile. *Hallucinations* are abnormal sensory perceptions in the absence of a stimulus (voices coming from a picture on the wall) while *illusions* are misinterpretations of stimuli (belief that the doorbell ringing is someone speaking). *Depersonalization* is the perception that one's body is strange and unreal, as though apart from the patient. *Derealization* is a similar perception of unreality and estrangement of objects in the environment.

Judgment and Insight

The student determines if the patient is realistic or unrealistic about his problem and other issues. An apparent obliviousness of a serious problem is called *la belle indifference*.

Neuropsychiatric Evaluation

1. The student observes the patient's level of consciousness (e.g., comatose, stuporous, drowsy, alert, hyperalert).
2. One carefully investigates attention and concentration by asking the patient to repeat a series of from three to eight digits (e.g., repeat the following: 8-1-6-3-9); having them subtract from 100 by 7 and continuing doing so with each answer, so-called serial 7s (e.g., $100 - 7 = 93$; $93 - 7 = 86$; and so on); spelling a word (like *world*) backward; and inquiring about immediate

occurrences in their environment (repeat the student's name after clearly stating it).

3. The interviewer also assesses the patient's language function for fluency, comprehension, naming, repetition, reading and writing. In addition to observing and listening to the patient, the student asks the patient to read and explain a simple text and to write a sentence or two on their own (without giving them the sentence); such exercises should be appropriate to the patient's level of education.

4. Recent memory is tested by determining the patient's orientation to time, place, and person; for example, the patient is asked to describe the day, date, year, time, place, and his name and identity. Recent memory also is tested by asking the patient to recall three objects immediately after mentioning them (e.g., comb, dog, the color yellow), then warning the patient they will be asked to recall the three objects in 3 to 5 minutes and, finally, testing the patient's recall at that time. Remote memory is evaluated by inquiring about events of several days earlier as well as events months and years earlier (e.g., "What day did you come into the hospital?" or "Who is the President?" or "What are your daughters' names?").

5. Other higher functions include how well the patient thinks abstractly. Interpreting proverbs such as "People who live in glass houses shouldn't throw stones," can vary from bizarre to very concrete to quite abstract and interpretive. Similarly, the student can determine the capacity for abstract thinking by inquiring how an apple and an orange are alike and different. Calculations and testing of general intelligence also can be helpful at times.

With most patients, one's usual interaction and observation constitute sufficient mental status evaluation and can confirm intact cognitive function. We routinely obtain full MSE in its entirety when we suspect dysfunction (of behavior, thought, or emotion) and in most new psychiatric and neurological patients. I advise medical students in beginning clinical clerkships to complete the full MSE in all new patient evaluations as a way of becoming familiar with it in normal and abnormal circumstances. Written reports of the patient should include comments on MSE in conjunction with the physical examination of the neurological system. Although mostly obtained earlier during the doctor-patient interaction, the MSE is part of the "physical examination" of the brain and its functional integrity.

A screening MSE may quickly detect cognitive dysfunction, and is useful when cognitive impairment is suspected [10]. In medical settings when there is suspicion of cognitive impairment, I suggest use of the mini-mental status examination (Fig. 6-1). This testing can be performed in 5 to 10 minutes and can help both diagnosis and follow-up of the course of cognitive dysfunction.

Pediatric Patients

Integrated Patient-Doctor Interviewing applies with children and adolescents as well as adults [12]. The interviewer still hopes to establish a relationship and obtain adequate personal and symptom data, but with emphasis on growth, development, and family interactions [13,14]. Relationship issues necessarily extend to parents and other family. The younger the child, the more age-related issues are involved: decreased ability to communicate, shorter attention span, less physical and mental development, and increased dependency on parents [13].

The usual conduct of steps 1–5 has to be modified in many pediatric patients, even some adolescents. Children often lack the psychological and physical maturity to participate fully at this level of independence and self-directedness, and the interviewer sometimes relies more on a doctor-centered process. Nevertheless, the child's concerns always are sought and we must recognize that children become increasingly autonomous as they grow older. It has been found equally important to directly involve our younger patients in treatment discussions and decisions [12]. The interviewer also uses a patient-centered approach in interacting with the parent, with a major focus on the child's problems.

The student continues to attend to the various steps of the interview, modifying the approach given the age and initiative of the patient. In step 1, age-appropriate opportunities and facilities are made available; for example, toys, chairs, games, and meeting the needs of teenagers who frequently do not want to sit with children or in childlike circumstances [13,14]. Older children and adolescents can often provide their own agenda, but parents usually formulate the issues for younger children [12].

The age of the child determines how steps 3 and 4 are best carried out. The interview involves the parent more when the patient is a

Fig. 6-1. The mini-mental status evaluation. Scores of 20 or less suggest further evaluation for organic cognitive dysfunction but also can be found in some psychiatric disorders. (Reprinted from Folstein MF, Folstein SE, McHugh PR. "Mini-mental state": A practical method for grading the cognitive state of patients for the clinician. *J Psychiatr Res* Copyright [1975], 12:189–198, with kind permission from Elsevier Science Ltd, The Boulevard, Langford Lane, Kidlington 0X5 1GB, UK.)

Patient _____

Examiner _____

Date _____

"MINI-MENTAL STATE"

ORIENTATION

Maximum Score	Score	
5	( )	What is the (year) (season) (date) (day) (month)?
5	( )	Where are we (state) (country) (town) (hospital) (floor)?

REGISTRATION

3	( )	Name 3 objects: 1 second to say each. Then ask the patient all 3 after you have said them. Give 1 point for each correct answer. Then repeat them until she/he learns all 3. Count trials and record.

Trials:

ATTENTION AND CALCULATION

5	( )	Serial 7s. 1 point for each correct. Stop after 5 answers. Alternatively spell "world" backwards.

RECALL

3	( )	Ask for the 3 objects repeated above. Give 1 point for each correct.

LANGUAGE

9	( )	Name a pencil and watch (2 points)

Repeat the following "No ifs, ands, or buts." (1 point)

Follow a 3-stage command:

"Take a paper in your right hand, fold it in half, and put it on the floor." (3 points)

Read and obey the following:

CLOSE YOUR EYES (1 point)

Write a sentence (1 point)

Copy design (1 point)

_____ Total score

ASSESS level of consciousness along a continuum

Alert	Drowsy	Stupor	Coma

Fig. 6-1 (continued)

INSTRUCTIONS FOR ADMINISTRATION OF
MINI-MENTAL STATE EXAMINATION

ORIENTATION

(1) Ask for the date. Then ask specifically for parts omitted, e.g., "Can you also tell me what season it is?" 1 point for each correct.

(2) Ask in turn, "Can you tell me the name of this hospital?" (town, county, etc.) 1 point for each correct.

REGISTRATION

Ask the patient if you may test her/his memory. Then say the names of 3 unrelated objects, clearly and slowly, about 1 second for each. After you have said all 3, ask the patient to repeat them. This first repetition determines her/his score (0–3) but keep saying them until she/he can repeat all 3, up to 6 trials. If the patient does not eventually learn all 3, recall cannot be meaningfully tested.

ATTENTION AND CALCULATION

Ask the patient to begin with 100 and count backwards by 7. Stop after 5 subtractions (93, 86, 79, 72, 65). Score the total number of correct answers.

If the patient cannot or will not perform this task, ask him to spell the word "world" backwards. The score is the number of letters in correct order, e.g., dlrow—5, dlorw—3.

RECALL

Ask the patient if she/he can recall the 3 words you previously asked him to remember. Score 0–3.

LANGUAGE

Naming: Show the patient a wristwatch and ask her/him what it is. Repeat for pencil. Score 0–2.

Repetition: Ask the patient to repeat the sentence after you. Allow only one trial. Score 0 or 1.

3-Stage Command: Give the patient a piece of plain blank paper and repeat the command. Score 1 point for each part correctly executed.

Reading: On a blank piece of paper print the sentence "Close your eyes," in letters large enough for the patient to see clearly. Ask her/him to read it and do what it says. Score 1 point only if the patient actually closes her/his eyes.

Writing: Give the patient a blank piece of paper and ask him to write a sentence for you. Do not dictate a sentence. It is to be written spontaneously. It must contain a subject and verb and be sensible. Correct grammar and punctuation are not necessary.

Copying: On a clean piece of paper, draw intersecting pentagons, each side about 1 inch and ask him to copy it exactly as it is. All 10 angles must be

Fig. 6-1 (continued)

present and 2 must intersect to score 1 point. Tremor and rotation are ignored.

Estimate the patient's level of sensorium along a continuum, from alert on the left to coma on the right.

Alert	Drowsy	Stupor	Coma

younger child. Even then, we should address the child first in an open-ended style and the child remains the focus of the inquiry [12,13]. The interviewer directly interviews children who can speak, irrespective of age, recalling their unfamiliarity with many medical and other words [12]. The younger the patient, the more concrete, simple, and brief the questions. One always tries an open-ended approach, sometimes productive even in the very young [13]. In fact, we often underestimate how much information we can get from little children (e.g., "Mommy says Daddy needs to get a better job"). Nevertheless, it frequently helps to initiate conversation by giving age-appropriate "menus" of topics to choose from [14]; for example, open-endedly inquiring about recent birthdays, school, siblings, athletic events, social events, friends, and the like. The interviewer's task is to get the child talking about whatever interests him. In addition, the interviewer wants to see children interact with the parent and others, perhaps observing them in the waiting room [13]. The student and child also interact, even if briefly, without the parent present. The student observes the child's behavior as well as his communication.

In steps 6 and 7 (HPI) the student obtains information from child, parent, or both in the fashion already described in Chapter 5. Step 8 (HI) and step 9 (PMH) require an additional emphasis. Because growth and development are critical, the younger the child the more detail is required about the mother's pregnancy, delivery, newborn and infancy periods, and subsequent deveopmental landmarks (e.g., feeding, growth, walking, talking, toilet training, progress in school, social development). Personal habits, immunization status, usual childhood illnesses, hospitalizations, poisonings, accidents, and injuries are biomedical data that merit special attention. As the child ages, the approach more closely resembles that of the adult PMH/HI.

Step 10 (SH) and step 11 (FH) also have unique foci. The SH contains information about the pertinent social aspects of the family (e.g., father's job) as well as the patient (e.g., less fighting at school and improved reading). The student inquires about salient family interactions as well (e.g., ignoring a new brother, parents getting along better since strike settled). It also has been helpful to speak with a child's teacher to best understand the SH, especially if the child is having problems.

The FH (step 11) includes the health histories of grandparents, parents, and siblings. Because genetic disorders and precursors of adult diseases frequently begin in childhood, the interviewer obtains a careful family pedigree. The mother's health is especially important and concerns menses, contraception, marriages, pregnancies and outcomes, subsequent progress of children, and plans for more pregnancies. The student also ascertains her feelings about her pregnancy with the patient, and learns about her physical and psychological health. Her own rearing (punishment practices, abuse) and expectations of what being and raising a child are like are germane. The student assesses what kind of mother she will be and looks for areas where an intervention may be helpful; for example, she may need support of her own competence. As mothers increasingly support families, their work situation is important as well. As fathers become more central to rearing children, many of the above considerations apply to them also. Indeed, fathers frequently are ignored and often feel left out at all levels of their child's care. They must be actively included and involved.

The student accords step 12 (ROS) more importance than with adults [14]. Because children have much shorter histories and because it can be more difficult to obtain pertinent symptoms during the HPI, detailed inquiry in all systems is made prior to physical examination and more attention is paid transient or "minor" complaints.

Adolescence is a tumultuous period physically and psychologically. A student must take this into account. Some adolescents will be perfectly comfortable with the standard patient-centered approach, while others can be made uncomfortable and anxious by this and benefit from a more structured, doctor-centered approach. Prominent issues and themes that can emerge are dependency on parents, being forced to come to the doctor, conflict with parents and others, confidentiality, desire to see an "adult doctor," obliviousness of health risks, hypochondriasis, mood changes, and rebelliousness [14]. Ordinarily, the interviewer begins with the patient-centered approach but is prepared to change to a more doctor-centered approach if the adolescent seems anxious or uncomfortable. It may be more important to provide support and comfort rather than obtaining open-ended information, particularly at the beginning of the relationship. Seeing the adolescent alone is often more effective and can lead to a better relationship.

Elderly Patients

While continuing to focus on the relationship and gathering data, geriatric patients also have unique issues the interviewer must address [7,15,16]. These are occasioned by multiple medical problems combined with greater functional, social, psychological, and economic impairment [7]. To understand and integrate this multiplicity of biopsychosocial problems, the student often must involve other professionals such as nurse, social worker, and therapist.

Setting the stage and ensuring comfort in step 1 requires special attention. The interviewer should consider the patient's comfort and pride (dentures available, full dress), their ease of hearing and seeing, and show proper respect (e.g., use surname). During the interview, many will tire if the pace is too fast and they don't have time to formulate their responses. The student checks frequently. In addition, friends and relatives may make the patient more comfortable and provide information; confidentiality issues of course must be clarified.

Agenda-setting in step 2 is difficult if there are many problems. Both doctor's and patient's time and the patient's fatigue may necessitate that the interviewer defer less pressing problems to a later visit; obtaining a full history may sometimes take two or three visits. Completion of a previsit history form (and sometimes other forms assessing functional status, mental status, and psychosocial status) can be useful adjuncts that provide necessary information without overly taxing the patient [7].

Steps 3 and 4 usually are conducted as already described. The following can sometimes greatly facilitate the interaction: touching the patient sensitively and caringly, showing interest and patience, and addressing the older person's priority items [7]. Because many patients are familiar with the medical system and know "what it wants," it can sometimes be difficult to get older patients talking on their own, rather than responding to questions. It may be hard to move them from physical symptoms to personal issues. Nevertheless, most respond to a patient-centered approach if the interviewer persists in its use.

Some older patients tend to recite long stories about the past, posing difficulty for the interviewer. Patients often tell "old war stories" to impress the student that they were, and therefore still are, people of value and dignity [7]. To shift the conversation, the interviewer must acknowledge what the patient is trying to say. For example, to a patient relating his successes with a job in 1949, the interviewer might say, "That's quite an accomplishment; you sure did a lot. We'll get back to that if we can, but let me shift gears and get you to say how things are going for you now."

The HPI/OCAP will be longer in most elderly patients because they usually have more than one problem, their multiple problems interact, and many problems are chronic with long histories. The student focuses primarily on currently active problems. Falls, painful feet and toes, incontinence, sexual dysfunction, waning memory, depression, insomnia, and decreased hearing and vision are common. Similarly, functional difficulties are increasingly common as people age: dressing, bathing, feeding, using the toilet, transferring, using a telephone, shopping, cooking, cleaning, driving, taking medications, and managing finances. Multiple losses (of spouses, siblings, and friends) and loneliness are prominent. There also may be more concerns about death and disability as well as about living circumstances and remaining independent.

Health issues (HI—step 8) are essential. We should not overlook the fact that elderly patients have active sexual interests and a high alcohol abuse rate. Health maintenance activities are important but frequently ignored; it is particularly important to make a nutritional assessment, not only for caloric excesses but also for deficiency. The student should make sure the patient has the opportunity to discuss advance directives and end-of-life issues. The past medical history (PMH—step 9) also is apt to be extensive. Once again, the interviewer focuses on problems relevant to the patient's health.

If not ascertained in the HPI/OCAP, the social history (SH/step 10) determines the patient's social situation and her support structure. As patients age, they may lose capacity in what was previously routine (e.g., bathing, cooking). It is essential, thereby, to learn specifically what their support structure is and how it is affecting their health (e.g., senior citizens' center, church groups, Meals on Wheels).

The family history (FH—step 11) can become quite complex and it is essential that only information still important to the patient's health be obtained; for example, a family history of elevated blood pressure or diabetes in an 80-year-old is of little value, but who is available to help is a critical question. Similarly, the review of systems (ROS—step 12) is addressed only to issues salient to the patient's health.

Unique Issues for the Student

How Much Time to Spend with Patients
Students at the start of the third year obtain complete histories from new patients, often inpatients. Beginning clinical students can ignore the need for efficiency. As experience accumulates, efficiency follows. Initially, the student takes at least 30 minutes with the patient-centered process of the HPI/OCAP (steps 1–5), and 2 or more hours in the remainder of the HPI/OCAP, HI, PMH, SH, FH, and ROS; physical examination will take another hour or more at the outset; students must carefully attend to the patient's comfort and sometimes may have to return at a later time to complete the evaluation if the patient tires. This is only the beginning. The student reads, discusses, synthesizes data, obtains data from other sources, plans and analyzes diagnostic interventions, participates in treatment decisions—and again interviews the patient.

By graduation, most students can conduct a full interview in 60 to 90 minutes and by completion of residency, in 30 to 60 minutes. New patients typically receive 1-hour appointments in residents' and advanced students' clinics. Follow-up visits with both inpatients (ward rounds) and outpatients (clinic visits) involve patients known to the doctor or student and ordinarily range from 5 to 30 minutes.

Audiotape Recording of Interviews
During initial instruction in patient-centered interviewing (steps 1–5), teachers will have introduced most students to audiotaping or videotaping, and students will have learned how to critique interviews. Because the interview is a core skill, clinical students are urged to continue taping interviews on their own. Self-critique and input from other students or faculty leads to continuing improvement.

Inexpensive audiotape recorders can be used with minimal inconvenience and great benefit. Students inform patients that taping is confidential and that the tape will be erased when its use is completed; patients should of course know if others will be listening to the tape and who they are. In getting permission to tape, one benefits from patients' usual willingness to help; for example, "Before we get started talking, I'd like to ask your help. I'm interested in improving my communication skills and would like to tape-record our interaction. I (and my instructor—or my group) will listen to it afterward to see how I could have communicated better. Nobody else will hear it. Then we'll erase it. It's sure nothing you have to do but would be a big favor to me." Patients rarely refuse. Steps 1 through 5 are especially important—to critique one's patient-centered skills and transition into the doctor-centered process.

Taking and Using Notes

During steps 1 through 5 (patient-centered process), the student unobtrusively can jot down a few pertinent words or dates. This helps when the patient is giving the chronology of her physical problem and can preclude the student asking about it during the doctor-centered process. Nevertheless, one avoids any excessive break in eye contact, disruption of information flow, or other hitch in the relationship. During the doctor-centered process, the interviewer almost always takes notes, sometimes quite extensive, but still keeps the primary focus on the patient.

Students frequently need to use notes themselves as reminders to recall all components of the HI, PMH, SH, FH, and ROS. Reminder notes, however, should be minimized during the patient-centered process.

The interviewer can explain the note-taking and ask the patient to give feedback if it interferes. For example, the student might say at the outset, "I'll be making an occasional note early on, and later I'll be taking more notes and using some of my own notes to refer to. This helps me get all the information about you and keep it in order. If that becomes disruptive for you, please let me know."

Clinical Conduct

Many of my students and residents have debated which behaviors and attitudes are appropriate and, in many discussions, generated the guidelines presented here. These suggestions are not intended to be comprehensive, however, and the student can add more.

The consensus has been that the following behaviors are the most important: unconditional positive regard, empathy, acting as the patient's ally, acting in the patient's interest, respect, self-confidence tempered with humility, encouraging patient autonomy without forcing it, recognizing at least one patient strength or unique attribute, awareness of the role of spirituality, being honest but hopeful, letting the patient know the student's role in his care and the student's reason for seeing him, introducing self and all others present, arranging a mutually satisfactory time to interact, attending to the patient's physical comfort before interviewing, anticipating issues that could disturb the patient, openly addressing confidentiality, providing service beyond the usual, and meeting specific requests from the patient.

My students and residents thought the following behaviors were seldom if ever appropriate when with the patient: smoking, drinking, or eating; chewing gum or a toothpick; swearing; behaving seductively or making sexual remarks or jokes; poor personal hygiene; uncomfortable joking or teasing; personal opinions about others; going beyond appropriate self-disclosure to discuss one's own problems; and making judgments that imply good or bad about the patient or others.

These discussions raised other difficult issues. While certainly wanting to avoid seductive behavior, what is the role of touching the patient outside the physical examination? The students and residents generally agreed that this was appropriate but only if it felt comfortable to the student or resident, was motivated out of genuine personal concern, and would appear professional. Although hugging or putting one's arm around a well-known patient can be appropriate and professional, they preferred more limited touching; for example, a pat on the back or arm.

We also puzzled over the conversation one conducts during the physical examination, especially during the more tension-laden portions; for example, pelvic, breast, or rectal examination. All agreed that calm, confident discussion of what one is doing and why is appropriate, of course attending to the patient's experience and comfort. Inquiry about symptoms and problems in the areas being examined also defuses tension. The interviewer can explain self-examination and other preventive techniques; for example, during breast examination, the student could instruct a woman in self-examination.

Summary

The interviewer makes key practical decisions during steps 1 through 5. These decisions guide the fine-tuning of the interview that is required for balancing the patient-centered and doctor-centered processes; for patients who are reticent, talkative, or focused on biomedical material; when all necessary personal data do not arise during the patient-centered process; when more than one person is present; with communication problems (deaf, mute, blind, cognitively impaired); and for pediatric and geriatric patients. Interviewing issues unique to the student include taking sufficient time for the interview, self-critique using audiotapes, the strategic use of notes at the bedside, and recommendations for appropriate clinical behavior.

References

1. Lipkin M, Putnam SM, Lazare A (eds.), *The Medical Interview*. New York: Springer-Verlag, 1995.
2. Beckman HB, Frankel RM. The effect of physician behavior on the collective of data. *Ann Intern Med* 101:692–696, 1984.
3. Campbell TL, McDaniel SH. Conducting a Family Interview. In Lipkin M, Putnam SM, Lazare A (eds.), *The Medical Interview*. New York: Springer-Verlag, 1995. Pp. 178–186.
4. Hardt EJ. The Bilingual Interview and Medical Interpretation. In Lipkin M, Putnam SM, Lazare A (eds.), *The Medical Interview*. New York: Springer-Verlag, 1995. Pp. 172–177.
5. Billings AJ, Stoeckle JD. *The Clinical Encounter—A Guide to the Medical Interview and Case Presentation*. Chicago: Year Book, 1989.
6. Enelow AJ, Swisher SN. *Interviewing and Patient Care*. New York: Oxford University Press, 1986.
7. Mader SL, Ford AB. The Geriatric Interview. In Lipkin M, Putnam SM, Lazare A (eds.), *The Medical Interview*. New York: Springer-Verlag, 1995. Pp. 221–234.
8. Leon RL, Bowden CL, Faber RA. The Psychiatric Interview, History, and Mental Status Examination. In Kaplan HI, Sadock BJ (eds.), *Comprehensive Textbook of Psychiatry* (vol. 1) (5th ed.). Baltimore: Williams & Wilkins, 1989. Pp. 449–462.
9. Andreason NC, Black DW. *Introductory Textbook of Psychiatry*. Washington, DC: American Psychiatric Press, 1991.
10. Folstein MF, Folstein SE, McHugh PR. "Mini-mental state": A practical method for grading the cognitive state of patients for the clinician. *J Psychiatr Res* 12:189–198, 1975.
11. Strain JJ, Putnam SM, Goldberg R. The Mental Status Examination. In Lipkin M, Putnam SM, Lazare A (eds.), *The Medical Interview*. New York: Springer-Verlag, 1995. Pp. 83–103.

12. Lewis C, Pantell B. Interviewing Pediatric Patients. In Lipkin M, Putnam SM, Lazare A (eds.), *The Medical Interview*. New York: Springer-Verlag, 1995. Pp. 209–220.
13. Greenspan SI, Greenspan NT. *The Clinical Interview of the Child* (2nd ed.). Washington, DC: American Psychiatric Press, 1991.
14. Enzer NB. Interviewing Children and Parents. In Enelow AJ, Swisher SN (eds.), *Interviewing and Patient Care* (3rd ed.). New York: Oxford University Press, 1986. Pp. 122–147.
15. Blazer D. Techniques for communicating with your elderly patient. *Geriatrics* 33:79–84, 1978.
16. Fletcher CR. How not to interview an elderly clinic patient: A case illustration and the interviewer's explanation. *Gerontologist* 12:398–402, 1972.

Doctor-Patient Relationship

Interviewing elicits information about the patient. In addition to the informational dimension, there is a second determinant of a successful interview—the doctor-patient relationship (DPR). Integrated Patient-Doctor Interviewing incorporates additional measures (beyond relationship-building skills) to better foster the DPR. This chapter addresses these determinants of the dyadic aspect of the DPR but does not consider more general determinants; for example, the sociocultural matrix, patients' and doctors' roles, and subcultures.

The DPR is a fundamental dimension of care; this relationship should be monitored as closely and continuously as the temperature, blood pressure, and pulse rate of the patient. To do this, we observe patients' body language, their behaviors, what they say and how they say it, how comfortable they are emotionally, and their ability to interact and negotiate. For example, a comfortable, safe, and otherwise healthy DPR is suggested if the patient's arms are not folded defensively across the chest, they make appropriate (intermittent) eye contact, they arrive on time and follow negotiated agreements, they openly express what concerns them including negative aspects of their care, they are comfortable expressing emotions including negative ones toward the interviewer, and they are able to negotiate solutions for their care. There are, of course, many variations. When the relationship is effective, patient and physician alike experience respect, trust, and an effective interchange of data. Both feel comfortable and note an increase in rapport, satisfaction, compliance, confidence, and openness to negotiation. The opposite features characterize an ineffective relationship.

To understand the dyadic aspects of the DPR, consider the doctor's personality and patient's personality as two interacting gears. The gears must engage to establish the relationship, lest we find ourselves in an uninvolved, distant interaction, perhaps wherein doctor and patient address different agendas. On the other hand, if the gears engage too deeply, the mechanism itself can be destroyed, resulting in overinvolvement of doctor and patient; for example, a sexual relationship. The student therefore must understand the patient's personality and his own personality. This understanding allows the interviewer to adjust his behavior so as to better mesh with the patient.

An Interviewer's Previously Unrecognized Responses Affect Her or His Relationship with the Patient

Because the patient cannot be expected to change, the student (and doctor) often must change to make the relationship most effective. Interviewers frequently exhibit personal responses that are counterproductive [1], and changing them improves the DPR. Most problems occur during steps 1 through 5 (patient-centered process) because the relationship is just beginning, and because it is here that the patient expresses most of the personal material that can be stressful to the student. Nevertheless, the interviewer's personal responses affect the doctor-patient relationship throughout.

I define a "personal response" as one's emotional reaction and its behavioral result. For example, a student became afraid of an authoritarian patient who reminded him of his father. This led him, in turn, to allow the patient to take over the interview, even though the interviewer knew better. Another interviewer became anxious and felt out of control when a patient began talking about sexual issues. This led her, in turn, to take excessive control of the interview by switching prematurely to the doctor-centered process. In each instance, the emotion (fear, anxiety) led to a nonproductive interviewing behavior.

Adverse emotions and behaviors can be triggered by any aspect of a patient; for example, personality, job, illness, family, or odor. Some doctors feel negatively about people with AIDS, perhaps due to unwarranted fears of catching it [2]; some about people abusing alcohol, often negative feelings about the patient's seeming unwillingness to take responsibility for their actions; and some about patients with no definable disease, often from frustration at the doctor's inability to make a disease diagnosis [3]. Negative feelings produce negative behaviors such as avoidance, criticism, or superficiality.

Deleterious emotions also can feel positive, as in the example already given of sexual attraction to a patient. Similarly, "liking" a patient because that patient reminds the student of a positive person in his life can be dangerous if the resulting behavior treats the patient as though the patient were that other person. This behavior ignores the patient's real self and needs; for example, avoiding discussion of cancer in an elderly woman who reminds the interviewer of her own much loved grandmother.

The Problem

Studies in medical students, housestaff, and fellows demonstrate that interviewers' responses to patients almost universally have negative components and deleterious potential. Thirteen of 15 sophomore medical students [4] and 16 of 19 residents and fellows [5] exhibited potentially harmful responses when observed in a single interview each. Table 7-1 lists the potentially deleterious feelings and their resulting behaviors. Common fears of losing control, of addressing psychological material, or of appearing unpleasant generate interviewing behaviors that are, respectively, overly controlling, avoiding of psychological material, and superficial. The student can imagine their harmful potential. Consider, for example, the life-threatening impact of avoiding data about suicidal intent, noncompliance, and specific symptoms—as well as the effect of these behaviors on data-gathering and the relationship itself.

A study of board-certified physicians with an average age of 50 showed that these doctors continued to exhibit potentially deleterious responses, particularly when threats to their integrity or self-esteem occurred [6]. While these seasoned practitioners reacted adversely to fewer patient circumstances than did students, residents, and fellows, their reactions did not diminish with age or experience. Once established, a pattern remains. This suggests that experience will not change potentially harmful behaviors unless we attempt specific educational interventions.

Troublesome unrecognized responses often override or interfere with new learning. Patient-centered practices entail relinquishing some control and addressing patients' emotional material but, because of strong personal responses, many interviewers act as if they wish to seize control and avoid emotions. Even though the student or resident demonstrates ability with newly learned patient-centered skills, long-ingrained emotions can interfere with using those very skills.

Table 7-1. Unrecognized feelings and resulting behaviors in students, residents, and fellows during one interview*

UNRECOGNIZED **FEELINGS** ELICITED IMMEDIATELY AFTER A PATIENT INTERVIEW

Common

Fears of: losing control, addressing psychological material, appearing unpleasant, harming the patient

Unique personal issues; e.g., reminds one of own difficult divorce, fear of cancer in self

Performance anxiety

Uncommon

Sexual feelings, attitude favoring biomedical data, anger, fear of involvement, intimidation by patient, inadequacy, disdain

Identification with the patient

Not found

Severe anxiety, depression

UNRECOGNIZED **BEHAVIORS** OBSERVED DURING A PATIENT INTERVIEW

Common

Overcontrol of the patient and interview; e.g., inappropriate interrupting or changing subject

Avoidance of psychological material; e.g., death, loneliness, disability

Superficial behavior; e.g., overly reassuring, overly social, cocktail party atmosphere

Passivity; e.g., no control or direction, inactive, detached

Uncommon

Seductiveness

Critical, intimidating, passive-aggressive

Lack of respect and sensitivity

Withdrawal, distancing

Awkward interactions

---

*These data were obtained by the author during and following training interviews. The author personally observed the learner-patient interview and noted untoward behaviors that were potentially unrecognized behaviors. The teaching critique followed immediately and always was begun with open-ended inquiry. This produced data about the learner's emotional response to the patient and also provided the data showing whether the interviewer was fully aware of the behaviors observed by the author. When the interviewer previously was fully aware of the emotions or behaviors observed by the author, they were not included; that is, only incompletely recognized emotions and behaviors are recorded here.

Adapted from Smith RC. Teaching interviewing skills to medical students: the issue of "countertransference." *J Med Educ* 59:582–589, 1984; and Smith RC. Unrecognized responses and feelings of residents and fellows during interviews of patients. *J Med Educ* 61:982–984, 1986.

What the Interviewer Can Do
About Unrecognized Responses

Unfortunately, most interfering responses are not fully conscious and therefore incompletely accessible to the interviewer. While effective coaching by a teacher [7] best helps one to become aware of previously unrecognized responses, the student can nevertheless make significant progress working alone or with colleagues [8].

Diagnosing the Problem

To diagnose difficulties with one's personal responses we must make our emotional responses more conscious and recognizable. The student can reexperience emotions by recalling negative or otherwise difficult experiences with patients, clinical situations, peers, and family. By thinking individually or talking freely with peers, the interviewer can become more aware and begin to understand his personal responses. First identify the emotion. Then link the emotion to a specific behavioral outcome; for example, the student was mad about a slight and ignored the provocateur. In considering many difficult situations, the interviewer usually finds a common pattern; for example, perceived slights provoked anger and withdrawal from nurses, friends, spouse, or a teacher.

Another exercise in better recognizing one's interfering emotions relates specifically to the interview. The first question following any interaction is, "What was my emotional reaction to the patient, and how did it affect my interviewing behavior?". The student can look for one positive and one negative emotion to each patient, and identify the behavioral responses. Consider imagined as well as actual behaviors; for example, wanted to spank a patient abusing alcohol "for being so stupid." Reviewing a video- or audiotaped interaction allows the interviewer to reexperience her emotional reactions and to more carefully observe for any untoward responses, such as unnecessarily changing direction or avoiding certain topics. Students who are not seeing patients can increase emotional awareness by considering other medical encounters: working on cadavers, operating on animals, having blood drawn, drawing blood, watching a discomforting procedure, reading about awful diseases, experiencing difficult contacts with teachers or peers, and the general medical school atmosphere. The student identifies the emotion and any behavioral consequence; for example, while observing a pelvic examination, the student became fearful it was causing pain, which led him to skip the next demonstration on pelvic exams.

There may be other routes to increase awareness of emotions. One can read emotion-laden material, watch emotional movies, recall personal emotional events, revisit music and art, work with emotional people, or consider likely emotional events in the future (births, deaths). One seeks positive as well as negative emotions. Other self-help or centering measures can be valuable to hard-working students and physicians. Increased calmness and poise usually help. One might try regular exercise, relaxation [9], meditation [10], taking personal time, nonintellectual pursuits, hobbies, creative endeavors, meeting different people, altruistic activities, and renewing the spiritual dimension.

Successful self-analysis and honesty go hand in hand [8]. It helps to realize that "negative" feelings are normal and universal [4,5]. We make things worse by ignoring them. Surprise awaits the student who believes emotions can be suppressed; there is always a consequence. For example, feeling angry at a patient or a peer will always have some behavioral consequence such as being too distant, overly friendly, or aggressive. Following an honest diagnosis of oneself, the student determines if the observed responses are taking her where she wants to be in her relationships. Once aware, the student can choose to change that response.

Treating Previously Unrecognized Behavior and Emotion

Repeatedly acknowledging the problem sometimes leads to improvement; for example, the student reminds himself before each interview that "discussing death and other painful issues is difficult and I need to be on the look-out." Usually, though, the interviewer must select a specific healthier behavior as a replacement, but not the ultimate, perfect behavior. Progressing a step at a time works better; for example, learning to make just a few comments is a good start for someone who has trouble talking in the presence of a professor. One rehearses the desired new behavior in mind and then in role play. In role play, with a peer, the student takes her own and then the other person's (or patient's) role in the problematic situation. She then reperforms both roles using the planned new behavior. This provides important reinforcement and insight about the old pattern and promotes satisfactory change in the new one.

Changing the emotion is more difficult. Sometimes self-supportive statements help; for example, "He just reminds me of my father. I have important things I want to say." Using emotion-handling skills with oneself helps. The student should consciously recognize that the work is uncomfortable, that he is working hard and trying new behaviors, and that progress, while slow, is occurring. The student reinforces her self-esteem with positive self-talk and recalls that this work will make her a better doctor [11,12].

Students can make remarkable changes as they get to know themselves better, take some risks, and stretch personally. Interviewers' innate capacity for adult growth and maturation uncovers unexpected strengths and capabilities that can lead to more effective relationships with patients—and others [13].

Doing this work with a few colleagues produces the best results. Others provide support, accurate feedback, and insightful suggestions for new behaviors. Within such groups (or pairs), the following are useful guidelines [14,15]:

1. Meet regularly for the sole purpose of self-awareness work.
2. Insist on strict confidentiality.
3. Urge people to speak only for themselves, and to participate only when ready and to the extent comfortable.
4. Direct feedback to focus on behaviors rather than the person; be sure the feedback is descriptive and nonevaluative, contains a balance of positive and negative, and provides only a manageable amount of information for the next step [16].
5. Focus on emotions and here and now events; intellectual discussions are appropriate but should not dominate.
6. Ask members not only to work with their own problems but also to try to be supportive and empathic to colleagues.
7. A nonjudgmental attitude and unconditional positive regard for each member keeps the setting safe and comfortable for the sharing that makes the process work.
8. Use predominantly open-ended questioning and remain person-centered.
9. Facilitate problem-solving and provide support: These are more valuable than advice, analysis, trying to change others, and "the hard truth."
10. Try to foster patience, understanding, and the recognition that each person's behavior is what works best for her or him; this offsets frustration with slow or inapparent progress. Many often do not understand or even recognize some very obvious aspects of themselves. Even after being addressed, the same issue often surfaces repeatedly and requires additional exploration.
11. Self-disclosure and responding to one's own emotions encourage others to do the same.

12. Recognize that respectfully and supportively discussing personal issues cannot harm another, and that others can take care of themselves; this assists in working with "painful" material.
13. Address feelings about other members of the group, especially when conflict occurs.
14. Always link personal issues and professional issues.
15. Expect to find that healthy, positive feelings often are among the most guarded and suppressed.
16. Realize that support leads to hope.
17. Appropriate touching helps, to the level of each member's comfort.
18. A facilitator can sometimes enhance the group's work. Seek help if problems or conflicts arise that interfere with the group work.

This process works even better if the student carefully analyzes his emotions and behaviors by keeping a journal or diary [15]. One synthesizes self-awareness work and identifies specific issues and behaviors to address in the future. Some useful guidelines for what to record are: most memorable events, most important learning, experiences applying new knowledge, emotions (and resulting behaviors), how behaviors have changed, how emotions have changed, specific new learning goals including the immediate next step, successes as well as problems, and whether the personal and group work are meeting expectations and why or why not.

A little anxiety and tension helps the student with this process, but she should not experience depression, marked anxiety, disruption of work or relationships, or other evidence of psychological disturbance. These outcomes require help from a mental health professional. It is noteworthy that self-awareness work does not "cause" problems but, rather, sometimes provides the forum for them to surface and, in turn, allows early identification.

Dimensions of the Patient that Affect the Relationship: The Patient's Personality Style

The patient's personality is far more difficult to change than one's own, nor should we try to do so. Nevertheless, a student who understands the patient's personality style can improve the relationship by adjusting his behavior to the patient's unique style. Personality style is defined as that group of enduring personal characteristics that describe how a person thinks, feels, behaves, and interacts in relationship to others and the environment [17–22]. Personality partially determines how people respond to the various stresses in life, including illness. It determines how the patient recognizes and presents his illness, how he relates to the doctor and nurses, how he will respond to treatments and procedures, how he deals with discomfort and disability, and how he will return to health and activity. Knowledge of a patient's personality alerts the interviewer to likely stressful circumstances that can perhaps be avoided or ameliorated. Designations of personality styles apply to doctors as well as patients. We can identify and name these styles but we must be careful to not use the terms pejoratively, as in name-calling or blaming.

Most personalities are within the range of normal, and readers will recognize parts of themselves in most styles described [17–22]. Moreover, styles usually are combined; for example, many people have both dramatic and organized styles. Personality characteristics are not just sources of trouble. They form the bedrock of psychological structure and are the basis of success as people make their way in the world; for example, a dramatic flair can be essential for a good performer or politician while an organized style is essential for an effective professional or a good homemaker.

One makes a psychiatric diagnosis (personality *disorder* in DSM-IV) only when the personality is maladaptive and interferes with successful functioning [21]; for example, overconcern about appearance that leads to mutilative procedures (numerous tatoos, unnecessary facial or breast reconstruction), or obsessively counting ceiling tiles and washing one's hands throughout the day. Maladaptive patterns can be precipitated or exacerbated in response to a medical illness. These patterns then may puzzle and obstruct physicians leading us to label the patient as "problem," "hateful," or "difficult" patients [23].

The interviewer can assess a patient's personality style during steps 1–5 and can use appropriate skills during this time based on her assessment of the patient's personality. She further diagnoses the style in step 4 by focusing on corroborating features and considering whether the style is adaptive or maladaptive. The sooner the patient's style is accommodated, the smoother the interaction.

This section describes how to enhance the relationship by using knowledge of the patient's personality style, comprehended from a constellation of features rather than from any one or two of them.

After identifying a personality style, the student meets the needs of its predominant feature to maximize the relationship. With normal, well-adapted patients this process is simply woven into each visit and the doctor proceeds as usual. Normal patients present no unique problems in the medical setting. Establishing the initial relationship with maladaptive patients, however, is just the start. These patients usually require ongoing care for this psychological problem, often by or in conjunction with a mental health professional, with a goal of developing more adaptive traits and gradually weaning patients from their maladaptive features. The student will note that each personality style has unique features that dictate different, sometimes opposite behaviors by the student.

Because this material is covered thoroughly during psychiatry rotations, only summaries of some major personality styles and how they affect the DPR will be presented here [17–22]. For illustrative purposes, maladaptive patterns (personality disorders) are emphasized, but one must remember that normal patients exhibit minor variations of these. Further, while this review presents each type singly, the reader will want to consider how different patterns might be combined. Most of us have features of several different personality styles.

Dependent Style

The basic problem in maladaptive dependent patients is an unconscious wish for boundless interest, attention, and care. Such attention represents love and assuages fears of abandonment, starvation, and helplessness that were learned very early.

Maladaptive patients, with naive expectations for endless love, reach out quickly and impulsively to doctors. They demand urgent, special attention, and behave as though no one else exists. The simplest instructions often require repetition and assistance; for example, how to get to the lab for a test. Losses and separations from loved ones are particularly stressful and can lead to illness and psychological deterioration. Because illness leads to caretaking, relinquishing its nurturing aspects when health is regained may be difficult.

The interviewer observes the following in better-adapted patients: normal and greater degrees of requests for advice, need for detailed directions, checking of plans in order to do things "right," "superindependent" behaviors wherein the patient delights in single-handedly performing many activities, living in the parental home as adults, deferring to a spouse for answers and decisions, using the collective "we" to indicate another's close involvement in their activities (e.g., "We took the medicine and then we did the physical therapy"), repeated stories of how others help and support them, and problematic oral habits (eating, smoking, drinking, addictions).

Maladaptive patients pose difficult problems in medical settings, becoming angry and frustrated when needs are not met. Incessant demands make the doctor feel "sucked dry." Many doctors who are mothers have likened the situation to having a child constantly tugging at their breast. Passivity, helplessness, and a sense of entitlement often preclude following directions, paying bills, and performing other responsible acts.

We can meet dependency needs during our initial contacts by incorporating much support into our conversation and actions; by evincing a positive outlook and showing interest in patients independent of disease; by giving guidance, advice, more detailed instructions, and special favors; and by arranging for more frequent visits.

Authoritarian interviewers typically interact nicely at the outset with dependent patients; for example, these doctors like to take charge and these patients like to be taken care of. Because maladaptive patients keep trying to get more and more, however, the doctor faces two possible relationship problems. First, he may try to meet the endless dependency needs so that the relationship becomes overinvolved, enmeshed, terribly time-consuming, and nonproductive. The doctor becomes frustrated from trying hard and failing, and the patient becomes frustrated in not getting enough. Second, the doctor may reject and distance himself from the patient so that the relationship dies.

Obsessive-Compulsive Style

The basic problem with maladaptive obsessive-compulsive patients is the unconscious need to maintain control, especially of emotional expression. Control assuages unconscious fears of emotion, dirtiness, disorderliness, impulsive aggression, and pleasurable indulgences—often the result of excessive childhood punishment.

Maladaptive patients use knowledge as a tool for controlling these fears. Thinking substitutes for emotion. Ritualistic behaviors and obsessive thinking replace action, and rationalizations are elaborate. Patients may bring extensive written notes for reference and give detailed, boring accounts of routine body functions and symptoms. Although asking many questions, they do not listen and obsessively focus on selected details as a way to control anxiety (rather than for intellectual need). Because illness bespeaks loss of control, they typically try to take control of medical interactions and often succeed. Obsessive patients guard against emotions. When asked how they feel or what their emotional reaction is, they characteristically respond with what they think.

The interviewer observes the following in better-adapted patients: normal and greater degrees of orderliness, precise speech, detailed information, self-discipline, tidiness, punctuality, conscientiousness, a well-organized approach, responsibility, conservatism, and concern with right and wrong.

Maladaptive patients in medical settings demand a great deal of time, having many questions and presenting detailed expositions of symptoms. Anger, depression, and anxiety may supervene when control falters. Self-doubt, indecisiveness, and vacillation can pose problems when medical decisions (especially urgent ones) have to be made.

Meeting an obsessive patient's needs means giving information in appropriate detail, which can include written material, and often must address specific plans for diagnosis and treatment. Repeated requests for information, however, indicate an underlying anxiety that must be explored rather than simply supplying information. It helps to involve the patient actively, giving her a sense of control in decision-making (e.g., which consultant to see) and in deciding the details of daily conduct (e.g., when blood is drawn, how bath will be given). The student puts the patient in charge, as long as it is comfortable to the patient and consistent with good care. Also, it may help to prominently compliment such patients on their knowledge, reasoning, self-sufficiency, and high standards.

Authoritarian interviewers can have trouble interacting with these patients if a battle for control ensues. This results in an unengaged relationship and patients may become unhappy and go elsewhere. If an authoritarian doctor yields appropriate control and gives information, the patient will be impressed by the doctor's remaining obsessive features such as thoroughness, precision, and clear reasoning.

Histrionic Style

The basic problem with maladaptive histrionic patients is the unconscious need to merge emotionally with others, especially of the opposite sex. Interacting in an emotionally intensive way gratifies, irrespective of the pain and discomfort it produces.

Maladaptive histrionic patients communicate through emotions, feeling, and performing rather than thinking and doing. They are overly dramatic, flamboyant, teasing, inviting, flighty, and impulsive. Concern about appearance and bodily integrity is paramount. Although histrionic patients can be quite personable, engaging, and entertaining at the outset, the interviewer soon notes a pervasive superficiality and lack of depth. Patients often are seductive in dress, style, and language. Women may present in a defenseless, vulnerable way or with sexual promiscuity. Histrionic men emphasize their manliness and courage before, and in the name of, women; plentiful tatoos, sexually revealing dress, and "macho" remarks are characteristic. Alternatively, men may present as effeminate, weak, and fragile. In the intellectual domain, maladaptive histrionics impress the interviewer as vague, imprecise, inconsistent, circumstantial, contradictory, and exaggerating. Such patients may have short attention spans, decreased ability to concentrate, and handle factual data erratically.

The interviewer observes the following in better-adapted patients: normal and greater degrees of charm, colorfulness, liveliness, attractiveness, sexual appeal, gregariousness, romanticism, sentimentality, artistic interest, and creativity. Many exhibit a zest for life and pleasure, have a rich fantasy life, and arouse the envy and admiration of others for these qualities.

Maladaptive patients in medical settings can become angry, depressed, and jealous if they are not noticed as attractive and outstanding. Dissatisfaction in the relationship can lead them, as it does in their personal lives, to precipitously leave for another caretaker. Their impulsivity and inexperience with sound reasoning leads to difficulties with drugs, medications, ill-advised surgery, and other decisions about care. Minor problems, especially perceived bodily defects, create ongoing anxiety. When deforming disease (breast surgery, facial laceration) occurs, these patients can be particularly vulnerable.

Meeting a histrionic patient's needs includes brief compliments on the patient's appearance made in a useful, tasteful, and nonsuggestive way. It is essential, however, to show and express interest in such a patient as a person rather than just as an object of attention. The interviewer behaves calmly and firmly when patients behave seductively. The interviewer allows patients to ventilate their fears and concerns, but does not foment or encourage them. Reassurance works better than intellectual explanations. One tries to involve these patients in decision-making, but the caretaker often must assist in the thinking process and not be reluctant to provide guidance, advice, and support.

To the extent the interviewer is susceptible to seduction or is seductive himself, these patients can prove disastrous. Sexual encounters between caretaker and patient are a harmful outcome of such interactions. Similarly, fears of such involvement can lead to the opposite—a distancing interaction. Most interviewers working with histrionic patients are troubled less by sexual issues, however, than by the patients' lack of sound cognitive skills, which can be a source of frustration to a more cerebral caretaker.

Self-Defeating (Masochistic) Style

The underlying problem with maladaptive self-defeating patients, a category whose existence as an entity has been questioned [21,24], is an unconscious need to suffer—probably resulting from a severely repressive upbringing (physical, sexual, or emotional abuse) that, nonetheless, symbolized love and attention. For example, if the child felt loved only when suffering or when the parent showed remorse following punishment.

Maladaptive patients repeatedly fail. Much suffering and bad luck, many disappointments, and a general hard-times impression typifies them. They present as the helpless victim, believing that they don't deserve success, and that if success occurs, something bad will follow to offset it. Such patients may precipitate their own misfortune and are often incapable of learning from prior mistakes, even when made aware of their repetitious patterns (e.g., the spouse of an alcoholic who repeatedly returns to the marriage or, once having left, finds another alcoholic).

The interviewer observes the following in better-adapted patients: normal and greater degrees of guilt and need to atone for misdeeds, complaining about their troubles, self-effacement and submission, expecting adverse outcomes, feeling unworthy of success, seeing themselves as victims without recourse, and meeting others' needs without concern for their own needs.

In the medical setting, maladaptive patients complain bitterly about many problems. Moreover, when one problem is resolved, they are not happy but, instead, present more difficulties. Reassurance typically leads to more complaints. There is resistance to encouragement, denial of improvement, accentuation of yet unimproved aspects of health, and a spurning of efforts to help. Patients frequently reject advice that would improve their situation (e.g., to quit riding a motorcycle that has caused five injuries). They often request painful procedures or surgery, and sometimes seek them out against advice.

In meeting these patients' needs, the interviewer avoids reassurance, suggestions of improvement, or promises of cure. Instead, the interviewer simply acknowledges and respects their plight. The emotion-handling skills work nicely for this. Certainly, one is never abusive to the patient, but tests or treatment can be framed as yet another burden. When patients exhibit a prominent martyr component, the interviewer frames interventions in terms of another's need.

These patients create a situation with great potential for an unwitting but nevertheless harmful interaction. They elicit much sympathy and caretakers respond by wanting to help, reassure, and cure. These responses are, however, counterproductive with self-defeating patients, create dissonance, and eventually lead to loss of the relationship and patient. Rather, the interviewer must restrain her usual more positive approach, acknowledge their plight, and provide a less hopeful, most austere atmosphere.

Narcissistic Style

The basic problem with maladaptive narcissistic patients is low self-esteem and lack of confidence in maintaining personal identity. To be intimate or accept anything from others means unconsciously merging with them and losing one's individuality. Narcissistic patients overcompensate by attempts to be superior and unique. This offsets low self-esteem.

Maladaptive patients present as all-powerful and all-important with an exaggerated self-confidence, often appearing smug, vain, arrogant, supercilious, possessing mysterious knowledge, disdainful of others' opinions, and grandiose. With others, they may be patronizingly superior, overbearing, callous, or aloof. Not surprisingly, they do not have close relationships, have difficulty establishing new ones, and are not described as friendly or warm. They irritate doctors, particularly by discoursing in prolonged monologues.

Working with better-adapted narcissistic patients, the interviewer observes the following: normal and greater degrees of expressing their opinions and feelings. The distinction between well-adapted and less well-adapted is whether this pattern represents a healthy self-respect and respects others' needs and opinions rather than representing an attempt to salve one's self-esteem.

In the medical setting, maladaptive narcissistic responses increase with illness; this is characteristically manifested by an attitude of superiority to physicians, always trying to "one-up" them, being content only with the "best" doctor (typically the Chief of Service), and being disdainful or patronizing of other physicians. In their incessant search for weakness in their caretakers, patients lose confidence as they dwell on the doctor's faults, thereby exacerbating their stress and narcissistic behaviors.

The interviewer meets the patient's needs by acknowledging the patient as a person of unique achievement, but at the same time is careful also to show expertise in a nonthreatening fashion, lest the patient lose confidence. It helps to engage the patient at medical levels by discussing recent journal articles and sharing ideas as one might with a colleague. The patient benefits most from an attitude of respect and concern rather than one of warmth and caring.

These patients often challenge or threaten authoritarian and other interviewers with their superior behaviors, lack of confidence, seeking out of other consultants, and ignoring of advice. The student may enjoy working with such a patient more if he can develop patience and not feel threatened.

Paranoid Style

The basic problem with maladaptive paranoid patients is an unconscious fear of their own faults, weaknesses, impulses (often retaliatory), and of infringement by others. These patients, often severely criticized as children, distrust others but remove their unwanted impulses by projecting them onto other people; for example, they see their own aggressive impulses in others. Their suspiciousness is rigid and intense, and characterized by a hyperalertness to anything out of the ordinary.

Maladaptive paranoid patients are guarded, vigilant, quarrelsome, suspicious, and fearful. They complain bitterly of mistreatment and neglect, and blame others for their problems. Oversensitivity to slights and alertness to the negative feelings of others are typical. They often feel persecuted and can respond with self-righteous counterattacks out of proportion to the magnitude of the perceived criticism.

The student observes the following in better-adapted people: normal and greater degrees of suspiciousness, critical evaluation, alertness to things out of order, cynicism, complaining, planning ahead to avoid dangerous circumstances, self-righteous statements, rigid limit-setting, ruminating on negative problems, and always anticipating problems.

In medical settings, a maladaptive patient's querulous approach for more attention, better food, less noise, faster nurses, and better clinic personnel is disrupting and time-consuming. Such patients, by threatening legal action and blaming others, frighten and irritate their caregivers. Anger and aggressive control of personnel engender an unhappy milieu. Depression and anxiety bespeak deterioration.

Meeting these patients' needs requires giving full information about plans and treatment, expecting to be more detailed than usual and subjected to greater scrutiny. The interviewer prevents inadvertent slights, including those by other staff. A friendly, courteous approach that avoids closeness works best. Attempts at more usual, closer relationships are met with great suspicion for what is perceived as an infringement. The interviewer does not reinforce, dispute, or ignore the patient's paranoid assertions. Rather, the student creates a sense of safety and acknowledges how difficult the problems are for a sensitive person like the patient to have to tolerate during an illness; one can also praise the patient's grasp of facts, self-control, and sense of autonomy. This, of course, is done using emotion-handling skills. One acknowledges feelings without either disputing or reinforcing them, and the patient is then ready for an appeal for more tolerance.

A paranoid patient creates considerable difficulty for authoritarian and other interviewers if they battle or ignore the patient. Even when these understandable tendencies are controlled, management is difficult and received without gratitude.

Schizoid Style

The basic problem with maladaptive schizoid patients is an unconscious fear of disappointment when relating to others. These patients may have experienced repeated early emotional deprivation and the absence of long-term ties (absent caretaker, erratic caretaking, multiple foster homes, institutional rearing) or the influence of schizoid or other distant parents—to make them uninvolved, detached, and remote. They never learned how to love or be loved. Aloofness is a protective denial of the many painful relationships gone awry.

Maladaptive schizoid patients isolate themselves. They are unsociable, out of touch, relate poorly, and have solitary interests. Although they may appear independent and not easily impressed, they often are oversensitive, fragile, and lacking in resilience. They frequently are of low socioeconomic status and using public support. Although usually uninterested, some have eccentric ideas and behaviors about foods, health measures, religious movements, social betterment schemes, and dress.

The student observes the following in better-adapted patients: normal and greater degrees of distance in relationships and comfort in being alone. Healthy people have relationships of varying degrees of closeness and involvement.

With maladaptive schizoid patients, illness threatens their seclusiveness and can occasion denial and minimization of severe, dangerous proportions. They may appear surprisingly undisturbed despite very significant problems. Typically, these patients are brought in by others, well-meaning relatives or neighbors. Solitary drinking is common but may go unrecognized. Patients are extremely poor on follow-up so that whatever needs to be done must be done initially. Compliance is poor.

Meeting schizoid needs means accepting the patient's unsociability and not threatening them with closeness or demands for relating. But the student does not permit withdrawal. This entails maintaining a considerate interest that is quiet and reassuring, and that does not demand reciprocation. One hopes to engage such patients to the degree they can tolerate although the relationships frequently remain distant and refractory to our best efforts.

Many physicians find these patients unappealing because of their inability to relate. Recalling their long-term deprivation helps the interviewer maintain steady but reserved interest.

Summary and Implications

The interviewer conducts steps 1–5 according to the guidelines outlined in earlier chapters. In addition, during steps 1 through 5 the interviewer identifies the personality style of the patient and then meets the unique needs, by matching her approach to the dominant patient style identified. This matching enhances the doctor-patient relationship by meeting deep psychological needs of the patient. This process works with normal patients, but maladaptive patients require even further efforts to develop healthier patterns, usually in consultation with a psychotherapist.

Even if changing a patient's personality to improve the relationship was possible, enormous amounts of time would be needed. Recent research does show, however, that patients' traditionally passive role can be changed to one of greater involvement to produce a better relationship and outcome [25–27]. This entails coaching patients to recognize relevant decisions and options, and encouraging more assertive behavior. Helping patients identify and formulate questions, rehearsing questions out loud, and developing strategies for negotiating decisions with the physician produce better health outcomes, and happier patients and doctors [25]. Systematic efforts requiring relatively little time and money could yield great dividends. For example, printed suggestions and illustrative videotapes could occupy patients in waiting rooms. A trained specialist could coach patients to formulate and rehearse questions, an approach that might be feasible where there are large numbers of patients waiting; for example, clinics, emergency rooms, admission offices.

Nonverbal Dimensions of the Relationship

Nearly all the material presented so far concerns the verbal aspects of interviewing. We now branch out to the nonverbal dimension and explore its powerful impact on the doctor-patient relationship (DPR) [28,29]. Prior to language acquisition, we all responded solely by nonverbal (bodily, somatic) means; for example, crying to express hunger or pain, smiling to express contentment [30–33]. With language acquisition, we acquired a new route for expressing emotion ("I don't like you, Mommie") [33]. However, the original capacity to experience and express emotion at a nonverbal level remains. Although normal growth and development requires that we integrate verbal and nonverbal expressions [31,34], much nonverbal material remains unintegrated [35,36] and nonverbal expression may remain incompletely recognized. This dissociation leads to the classic mixed message [28]; for example, a patient answers "yes" to a request to stop smoking while shaking his head in a negative way. The savvy interviewer knows this represents ambivalence.

Nonverbal responses give the interviewer a picture "beyond words"; for example, seductive, angry, or depressed. By integrating nonverbal and verbal information during the interview, the interviewer gets a better picture of the whole person. In this way the interviewer most fully understands the patient and her suffering, and makes the most meaningful connection possible.

Ensure Conducive Spatial Arrangements

By paying attention to the geography of the interview room, an interviewer ensures that the spatial arrangement promotes the relationship. For example, the interviewer should not sit or stand higher than the patient [35]. When dealing with a very ill patient lying supine or with a child, the interviewer can sometimes reduce the disparity by sitting down. The interviewer empowers rather than overpowers [35]. The interviewer also tries to avoid barriers, such as a desk, between himself and the patient, and to work at an optimal distance, neither too close nor too far.

Observe Systematically for Nonverbal Cues

To observe the patient's nonverbal expressions, it may help to consciously tune out verbal material briefly, as though watching television without the sound, and systematically look for nonverbal data. Nonverbal cues, as outlined in Table 7–2 [36,37], interact to characterize many of the emotions in Appendix A. The student might consider what nonverbal cues characterize each emotion listed; that is, what unique somatic or nonverbal features typify anxiety, grief, despair, joy, love, devotion, and determination? From the other direction, what is a possible emotional meaning of the following commonly observed nonverbal responses: leaning away from the interviewer; frequent patting or stroking of the interviewer's hand, arm, or knee; quivering lower lip; arms tightly crossed over chest; frown; slumped shoulders; furrowed brow; standing to talk; glistening of eyes (tearing); or smiling. As reviewed in Chapter 3, the student also will want to integrate other nonverbal data concerning physical characteristics (emaciated), autonomic changes (sweaty palms), accoutrements (tattered clothing), and environment (no greeting cards).

As early as the initial conversation of step 1, the interviewer begins to consciously observe the patient's emotional responses. This gives an idea of the patient's associated nonverbal response pattern and lets the interviewer recognize them more easily later on [35].

To this point, we have observed and interpreted nonverbal behaviors, but done little about them. Now we will begin working with nonverbal material.

Pacing, Matching

Pacing is a neurolinguistic programming concept wherein the interviewer subtly matches a patient's nonverbal expressions to

Table 7-2. Categories of nonverbal communication

Category	Includes	Examples
Kinesics (body language)	Body position (angulation, tension) Gestures Posture Gait Facial appearance	Leaning forward tensely with chin projected Making a fist Tip-toeing walk Depressed facies Tearing of the eyes
Touching	Handshake Other touching, including during physical examination	Weak handshake Overpowering handshake Seductive pat on arm
Paralanguage (everything but content of language)	Rate and rhythm of speech Voice pitch Inflection Volume Sighs and grunts Tone of voice Pauses	Rapid and jerky voice Low-pitched voice Peculiar inflection Very loud voice Frequent sighing Fearful tone No pauses
Spatial	Vertical and horizontal distance to another Angles of facing each other Physical barriers in the space	Doctor standing over a supine patient Far-removed interaction Desk between two people

Adapted from Levinson D. *A Guide to the Clinical Interview.* Saunders, 1987. Pp. 135–145; and Carson CA. Nonverbal communication in the clinical setting. *The Cortlandt Consultant,* Feburary: 129–134, 1990.

establish unconscious rapport [35,38,39]. The student mirrors the patient slowly to avoid distracting or alarming her; for example, observing that a patient had her head tipped to one side, the interviewer would slowly adopt a similar position; with a patient who gestured a lot with his hands, the interviewer would slowly begin similar hand gestures; talking to a patient who frequently pursed her lips, the interviewer might emulate this unobtrusively. Pacing applies to a vast range of behaviors, especially those in the kinesics and paralanguage categories of Table 7-2. Pacing need not be complex and can be as simple as mirroring the way the patient crosses his legs, folds his arms, or rubs his chin.

Leading

People in nonverbal synchrony with others may want to stay there. A leading behavior by one member induces a reciprocal act by the other, as long as it is introduced slowly and subtly [35,38,39]. This provides two opportunities for the interviewer [35,36]: (1) if the patient follows a lead, it confirms nonverbal connectedness; (2) to lead the patient away from nonproductive behaviors; for example, after matching a patient's persistent frown, the interviewer might gradually introduce a slight smile, hoping that the patient will follow the gesture and indeed feel better.

Addressing Nonverbal Behaviors

The interviewer addresses overt nonverbal expressions of emotion with emotion-handling skills (NURS; see Chap. 2); for example, to a crying patient, "That's really sad for you and I can understand. . . ." With less overt nonverbal messages, one relies on emotion-seeking and focused open-ended queries, and focuses on the nonverbal behavior; for example, "You look a little down, how do you feel about that?" or "You seem kind of tense," or "You look like the cat who swallowed the canary." This deepens the story and the doctor-patient relationship. Sometimes the student just notes but does not address the nonverbal behavior if she suspects that addressing the behavior would be poorly timed or offensive; for example, one often does not address the fact that the patient's arms are tightly folded across the chest in a defensive way.

Mixed messages represent conflict, perhaps conflict with the doctor, that must be explicated if communication and the relationship are to be maximized. The following can be helpful [35,36]. (1) Indirectly acknowledge the disparity; for example, to a patient saying work was great who, at the same time, is shaking his head negatively, "I hear what you say but I still get the feeling that things aren't going too well at work." If this prompts appropriate, congruent discussion, no more is necessary. One also might frame the incongruity in terms of a third person; for example, "I know some people in your work situation where difficulties arose and they were concerned about their jobs." (2) Sometimes, the student addresses the incongruity directly, although one usually has to know the patient well enough to be comfortable that their action will not be perceived as mocking; for example, a student says, "I notice you saying 'all is well' but shaking your head 'no.' What about that?" Interviewers themselves often send mixed messages; for example, "I'd like to hear more about that" while standing up to leave. The interviewer should try to avoid sending mixed messages such as this.

Summary

Facility with the informational aspects of Integrated Patient-Doctor Interviewing, presented in Chapters 1–6, goes only part way. Maximal flexibility and adaptability requires new skills with the more unconscious, interactional aspects of interviewing. Conducting the interview and experiencing patients as human beings often creates untoward responses that then produce harmful effects on the relationship and communication. The student improves the doctor-patient relationship by vigorously pursuing self-awareness and changing her or his own undesirable responses. In addition, patients' presentations and responses vary as a result of their unique personalities. The effective interviewer must recognize these styles and interact according to the personalities' unique dictates. Finally, the interviewer enhances communication and the DPR by recognizing patients' nonverbal emotional expressions and responding to nonverbal as well as verbal cues. Facility with DPR skills brings the relational dimension to equality with the informational, and provides the "second determinant" of a good interview. Because the student incorporates relational skills within a structure already present, the interview takes little additional time.

References

1. Brody H. *The Healer's Power*. New Haven: Yale University Press, 1992.
2. Epstein RM, et al. Understanding fear of contagion among physicians who care for HIV patients. *Fam Med* 25:264–268, 1993.
3. Ford CV. *The Somatizing Disorders: Illness As a Way of Life*. New York: Elsevier Biomedical, 1983.
4. Smith RC. Teaching interviewing skills to medical students: The issue of "countertransference." *J Med Educ* 59:582–589, 1984.
5. Smith RC. Unrecognized responses by physicians during the interview. *J Med Educ* 61:982–984, 1986.
6. Smith RC, Zimny G. Physicians' emotional reactions to patients. *Psychosomatics* 29:392–397, 1988.
7. Smith RC. Use and Management of Physicians' Feelings During the Interview. In Lipkin M, Putnam SM, Lazare A (eds.), *The Medical Interview*. New York: Springer-Verlag, 1995. Pp. 104–109.

8. Reik T. *Listening With The Third Ear: The Inner Experience of a Psychoanalyst*. New York: Farrar, Straus & Giroux, 1948.

9. Benson H. *The Relaxation Response*. New York: William Morrow, 1975.

10. Kabat-Zinn J. *Wherever You Go, There You Are: Mindfulness Meditation in Everyday Life*. New York: Hyperion, 1994.

11. Wood JT. *The Little Blue Book on Power*. Winslow, WA, 98110: Zen 'n' ink, PO Box 11714, 1990.

12. Stone H, Stone S. *Embracing Your Inner Critic*. San Francisco: Harper, 1993.

13. Erikson, EH. *Childhood and Society* (2nd ed.). New York: WW Norton, 1963.

14. Yalom ID. *The Theory and Practice of Group Psychotherapy* (3rd ed.). New York: Basic Books, 1985.

15. American Academy on Physician and Patient: Standards Document. Mack Lipkin, Jr., MD, NYU Medical Center, Dept. of Medicine, 550 First Ave., New York, NY 10016. (Document available upon request.)

16. Ende J. Feedback in clinical medical education. *JAMA* 250:777–781, 1983.

17. Shapiro D. *Neurotic Styles*. New York: Basic Books, 1965.

18. Kahana RJ, Bibring GL. Personality Types in Medical Management. In Zaiberg NE (ed.), *Psychiatry and Medical Practice in a General Hospital*. New York: International University Press, 1964. Pp. 108–123.

19. Lipkin M. The Medical Interview and Related Skills. In Branch WT (ed.), *Office Practice of Medicine*. Philadelphia: Saunders, 1987. Pp. 1287–1306.

20. Andreasen NC, Black DW. Personality Disorders. In Andreasen NC, Black DW (eds.), *Introductory Textbook of Psychiatry*. Washington, DC: American Psychiatric Press, 1991. Pp. 333–354.

21. American Psychiatric Association: *Diagnostic and Statistical Manual of Mental Disorders* (4th ed.). Washington, DC: American Psychiatric Association, 1994.

22. Putnam SM, et al. Personality Styles. In Lipkin M, Putnam SM, Lazare A (eds.), *The Medical Interview*. New York: Springer-Verlag, 1995. Pp. 251–274.

23. Groves JE. Taking care of the hateful patient. *N Engl J Med* 298:883–887, 1978.

24. Skodol AE, et al. Validity of self-defeating personality disorder. *Am J Psychiatry* 151:560–567, 1994.

25. Kaplan SH, Greenfield S, Ware JE. Impact of the Doctor-Patient Relationship on the Outcomes of Chronic Disease. In Stewart M, Roter D (eds.), *Communicating with Medical Patients*. London: Sage Publications, 1989. Pp. 228–245.

26. Shear CL, et al. Provider continuity and quality of medical care—a retrospective analysis of prenatal and perinatal outcome. *Med Care* 21:1204–1210, 1983.

27. Egbert LD, et al. Reduction of postoperative pain by encouragement and instruction of patients—a study of doctor-patient rapport. *N Engl J Med* 270:825–827, 1964.

28. Feldman SS. *Mannerisms of Speech and Gestures in Everyday Life*. New York: International Universities Press, 1959.

29. Larsen KM, Smith CK. Assessment of nonverbal communication in the patient-physician relationship. *J Fam Pract* 12:481–488, 1981.

30. Rodin G. Somatization and the self: psychotherapeutic issues. *Am J Psychother* 38:257–263, 1984.

31. Barsky AJ, Klerman GL. Overview: hypochondriasis, bodily complaints, and somatic styles. *Am J Psychiatry* 140:273–283, 1983.

32. Katon W, Kleinman A, Rosen G. Depression and somatization: a review (part 1). *Am J Med* 72:127–135, 1983.

33. Stern DN. *Diary of a Baby*. New York: Basic Books, 1990.

34. Engel GL. *Psychological Development in Health and Disease*. Philadelphia: Saunders, 1962.

35. Carson CA. The Hidden Language of Medicine: Nonverbal Communication in Clinical Encounters. Unpublished manuscript; Dept. of Medicine, The Genesee Hospital, Rochester, NY.

36. Carson CA. Nonverbal communication in the clinical setting. *The Cortlandt Consultant* February: 129–134, 1990.

37. Levinson D. *A Guide to the Clinical Interview*. Philadelphia: Saunders, 1987.

38. Bandler R, Grinder J. *Frogs Into Princes: Neuro Linguistic Programming*. Moab, Utah: Real People Press, 1979.

39. Christensen JF, Levinson W, Grinder M. Applications of neurolinguistic programming to medicine. *J Gen Intern Med* 5:522–527, 1990.

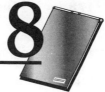

Presenting the Patient's Story

The student has generated a database of symptoms and personal issues, translated it to a biopsychosocial story about a human being and his illness, and worked to create an effective doctor-patient relationship. Now what? How does she now summarize and transmit this information to others?

Summarizing the Patient's Story

Even if the student has gathered a great deal of information and has synthesized it sensibly, there remains the task of meaningfully summarizing to reflect the essence of the patient—his biopsychosocial story, which includes disease diagnoses [1]. Our proposed multidimensional scheme integrates mind (psychosocial) and body (biomedical) components to describe the whole person and her dynamically interacting parts.

There are three components of the patient's biopsychosocial description: **R**elationship story, **P**ersonal story, and **D**isease story/diagnoses (RPD). These are outlined in Table 8-1, and illustrated at the end of this chapter and at the end of Appendix B where Mrs. Jones' story is summarized.

Relationship Story

The interviewer's experience during the entire interview allows him to synthesize a story of the doctor-patient relationship, which some believe to be the most central feature of medicine, called relationship-centered care [2]. Students often can be as successful as practitioners in this domain because the cardinal skill seems to be facility with personal self-awareness.

Table 8-1. Components of the patient's biopsychosocial story*

Relationship Story
  1. Interviewer's responses
  2. Patient's personality
  3. Doctor-patient interaction
Personal Story
Disease Story (Diagnoses)
  1. Biomedical
  2. Psychiatric

*The mnemonic RPD aids in remembering these components (see bold). The interactions of each component are usually given as part of the personal story.

Interviewer's Responses

The interviewer first needs to sort out and be conscious of personal feelings and resulting behaviors, occurring any time in the interview, toward the patient or the patient's circumstance; for example, fear of harming the patient that could lead to avoiding discussion of death, abhorrence of the patient's grotesque eye injury leading to unexplained trembling, fear of catching AIDS leading the student to avoid touching the patient, or feeling sexually attracted to the patient leading to excessive attention. As noted in the later examples, the student protects her own confidentiality and publicly expresses (in a written report or verbal presentation) only material that they are comfortable having many others know; more personal material is neither written nor presented and is reserved for discussion with preceptors.

Patient's Personality

The student makes his observations throughout the interview and identifies the patient's dominant personality style as dependent, histrionic, obsessive, self-defeating, narcissistic, paranoid, or schizoid (or other types), as outlined in Chapter 7. For most people, this designation depicts only their style of interacting with others. When personality style interferes with normal functioning, however, it is called a personality disorder [3].

Doctor-Patient Interaction

Finally, the interviewer must consider the interactional process itself and note any difficulties. Does the interview feel strained? Is there a nice give and take? Is the interview formal, collegial, parent-child, conflicted, competitive, or charged?

Personal Story

Synthesis of the multiple bits of the personal data, often gathered largely during the patient-centered process, produces a psychosocial story or theme. This ordinarily is quite straightforward. Students can identify the major issues and summarize them in two or three sentences. While every patient is unique, the following themes occur frequently [4]:

1. fear of death, mutilation, and disability;
2. dislike, distrust, and disbelief of the medical system and physician;
3. concern about loss of function, wholeness, role, status, and independence;
4. denial of problems;
5. separation, grief, and losses of many varieties;
6. leaving home and becoming independent;
7. retirement;
8. marital or job problems;
9. other unique personal problems of the patient; and
10. administrative issues relating to the disease diagnosis (e.g., requesting disability).

Disease Story

Similarly, the student synthesizes multiple bits of primary and secondary data to make disease diagnoses or, at least, high-level designations of the disease problem. A list of problems or diagnoses represents the disease story. Such a list usually numbers 3 or 4, but there can be as many as 15 or 20 problems/diagnoses in complex patients. Data for problems and diagnoses derive from the personal description of symptoms during the patient-centered process and their further clarification during the doctor-centered process and the physical examination. Of course, more knowledge of disease patterns makes it easier for clinical students to make diagnoses (e.g., angina or infectious hepatitis). Preclinical students, however, are not expected to make diagnoses and simply describe and list the problems identified and characterize them as fully as possible; for example, chest pain occurring with exercise and relieved by rest, vomiting and jaundice of recent onset where one other family member has the same problem.

Biomedical

The following are a few of the disease diagnoses common in adult nonpsychiatric settings, although they may not always be identified after only one interview and physical examination: hypertension, arteriosclerotic heart disease, diabetes mellitus, chronic bronchopulmonary disease, osteoarthritis, dermatitis, hypothyroidism, muscle strain and sprain, otitis media, upper respiratory infection, infectious sore throat and diarrhea, cataracts, glaucoma, acid peptic disease and gastritis, hemorrhoids, colonic polyps, urinary tract infection, cystitis, benign prostatic hypertrophy, prostatitis, sexually transmitted diseases, endometriosis, dysfunctional uterine bleeding, trichomoniasis, migraine, stroke, neuritis, radiculopathies, drug reactions, and health maintenance problems (e.g., elevated cholesterol). See below for common psychiatric problems that present in nonpsychiatric settings.

Even after thorough clinical and laboratory evaluation, many patients do not have a satisfactory disease explanation for their physical symptoms. Sometimes symptoms clear and we never know what caused them. Occasionally, symptoms persist and patients are later found to have a disease. Many of these patients, though, are designated by the general term *somatization* by which we mean an unconscious process wherein patients express emotional distress via physical symptoms.

Psychiatric

Over 50 percent of all psychiatric patients are seen only in a medical setting [5] and 20 to 25 percent of medical patients have a psychiatric diagnosis [6]. These psychological diagnoses and problems include depression, anxiety, adjustment disorders, addicting behaviors (tobacco, caffeine, alcohol, drug), homelessness, and abuse (psychological, sexual, physical—often involving elderly, children, spouses).

How do the relationship story, the personal story, and the disease story interact? How does the interviewer describe them to others? I suggest describing this interaction primarily with the patient's personal story, where one notes how it interfaces with disease diagnosis and the doctor-patient relationship. Interactions also can be recorded in the disease and relationship categories.

The American Psychiatric Association has published a compendium of all psychiatric diagnoses in its Diagnostic and Statistical Manual of Mental Disorders (DSM-IV) [3]. DSM-IV served as a conceptual basis and guideline for the RPD scheme presented in this book. DSM-IV categorizes patients on the following five axes: (1) psychiatric diagnosis, (2) personality disorder, (3) general medical condition (physical diseases), (4) psychosocial and environmental problems, and (5) global assessment of functioning in the past year. The first three dimensions overlap somewhat with the RPD classification. The five-axis approach in DSM-IV seldom is used in medical settings and I recommend it only after students have learned more clinical psychiatry. Students will find the RPD categorization easier since it includes elements pertinent to medical settings: the patient's personal story, the doctor-patient relationship, and the student's feelings. Either multidimensional scheme improves markedly upon a limited biomedical list of diseases [1,7].

The interviewer needs to first identify and then update the RPD. By frequently returning to the RPD designation, the interviewer can decide which diagnostic area needs the most attention. The student cannot put the story to rest as a fixed event or unchanging "reality." The story changes as diagnoses are resolved, as treatment is implemented, as new personal responses occur, and as the relationship deepens. Indeed, the very telling of the story leads to new thoughts and emotions about oneself and, in turn, to new actions and attitudes so that a new, different story evolves as part of the narration process [8–11].

The Medical Record:
Writing Up the Patient's Story

In the next step, the student records information in the medical record, notorious for omitting most psychosocial data [7]. This written description is usually called the *write-up* and is presented in the following outline. Appendix B contains a full write-up of Mrs. Jones' initial evaluation.

Recording the New Patient Evaluation: The Write-Up
1. Identifying data: age, gender, job, race, marital status, immediate family status, address, telephone number of nearest relative in case of emergency, referral source (if any)
2. Source and reliability of information: patient, relative or translator (specify), outside records (indicate completeness), judgment of reliability of information from all sources
3. Chief complaint and agenda: the patient's most bothersome complaint and a summary (list) of all presenting complaint(s)
4. History of present illness (HPI) and other current active problems (OCAP)

a. Overview of symptoms and time of onset
b. Complete description of the dimensions of each symptom; i.e., location, quality, quantitation, chronology and timing, setting, moderating factors, and associated symptoms
c. The absence of pertinent symptoms
d. Relevant positive and negative secondary data
e. The personal contextual dimension of the above; e.g., story content, emotions, patient's beliefs and explanations, impact of illness on daily life, relationships, support systems, practical issues, and role of stress

5. Health issues
a. Ethical-social-spiritual issues: advance directives, living will, "do not resuscitate" wishes, power of attorney, whom to contact if the patient cannot speak for her/himself, and spiritual practices
b. Functional status: dressing, bathing, feeding, transferring, walking, shopping, using the toilet, using the telephone, cooking, cleaning, driving, taking medications, managing finances, and cognitive function; extent of interference with normal life
c. Health-promoting and health-maintenance activities
   (1) Health promoting habits: diet, seat belts, use a helmet when riding a bicycle or motorcycle, protection of self and others from poisonous substances (including medications) and dangerous circumstances at home and at work, exercise, relaxation, recreation
   (2) Health screening: periodic health exams, mammograms, Pap smear, sigmoidoscopy, stools for occult blood, cholesterol, blood sugar, serologic test for syphilis, tuberculosis skin testing, HIV testing, prostatic evaluation, dental check, audiograms, eye exam, tonometry; self-examination (breasts, genitals, and skin)
   (3) Disease prophylaxis: diphtheria, pertussis, tetanus, polio, measles, German measles, hepatitis, influenza, vaccine for pneumococcal pneumonia, for diseases in areas of foreign travel
d. Health hazards
   (1) Use of addicting substances: caffeine, tobacco, alcohol, street drugs, prescription medications

        (2) Sexual practices: activity, preferences, diseases, abuse, risky habits, contraception, satisfaction

        (3) Abuse: sexual, physical, verbal, psychological, other

6. Past medical history

  a. Hospitalizations: surgical, nonsurgical, psychiatric, obstetric, rehabilitation, other

  b. Other medical, surgical, or psychological problems: childhood illnesses (mumps, measles, German measles, chicken pox), injuries, accidents, illnesses, unexplained problems, procedures, tests, psychotherapy, other

  c. Screen for major diseases: rheumatic fever, diabetes mellitus, tuberculosis, venereal diseases, cancer, heart attack, stroke; major treatments in the past (cortisone, blood transfusions, insulin, digitalis, anticoagulants); and visits to the doctor during the last year

  d. Medications and other treatments: prescribed, over-the-counter, alternative therapies and health care, and "non-medications" (laxatives, tonics, hormones, birth control pills, vitamins)

  e. Allergies and drug reactions: allergic diseases (e.g., asthma, hay fever), drugs, foods, environmental

  f. Menstrual and obstetric history (for women): onset of menses, duration, cycle length, discomfort, number of pads or tampons daily, birth control pills and other hormonal preparations, pregnancies, abortions (spontaneous), abortions (induced), deliveries of living children, other deliveries, complications of pregnancy

7. Social history

  a. Current personal situation

        (1) Demographic: age, sex, race, current work and living situation

        (2) Impact (meaning) of illness on self and others

        (3) Beliefs/explanations about illness

        (4) Relationships and support system

        (5) Practical issues

        (6) Stress

        (7) Financial situation

  b. Other personal factors

        (1) Early developmental outline: birth and early development, early family setting and other caretakers, relationship with parents and siblings, others' in-

teractions in family, early schooling and progress, places of residence, major losses and other adverse events, medical-surgical problems, happy events, later education and progress, social life and relationships, dating, adolescence, military or other service, getting away from home

(2) Marriage/other relationships and outcome: significant relationships (origin, course, outcome), children

(3) Work history and outcome: jobs and duration, satisfaction, toxic or other dangerous exposure (fumes, radiation, noise, dusts, chemicals)

(4) Recreational history

(5) Retirement

(6) Aging

(7) Life satisfaction

(8) Cultural/ethnic background

8. Family history

a. General inquiry

b. Inquire about specific diseases or problems: tuberculosis, diabetes, cancer, heart disease, bleeding problems, kidney failure or dialysis, tobacco use, alcoholism, weight problems, asthma, and mental illness (depression, schizophrenia, multiple somatic complaints)

c. Develop a genogram

(1) Two generations preceding the patient and all subsequently; involves parents, siblings, children, and significant members outside the bloodline for each generation

(2) Age, sex, mental and physical health, and current status are noted for each; note age at death and cause

(3) Note interactions among family members for psychological and physical problems

(a) Psychological

(i) dominant members and their style (e.g., loving, angry)

(ii) major interaction patterns (e.g., competition, abuse, open, distant, caring, manipulation, codependent)

(iii) family gestalt (e.g., happy, successful, losers)

(b) Physical
  (i) patterns of disease (e.g., dominant, recessive, sex-linked, no pattern)
  (ii) patterns of physical symptoms without organic disease (e.g., bowel trouble, uncoordinated, flighty)
  (iii) inquire about others with similar symptoms (e.g., infection, toxicity, anxiety, anniversary reaction)
9. System review of items not already considered: review of systems (ROS)[a]
  a. General symptoms
     (1) Poor appetite
     (2) Excessive appetite
     (3) Weight loss
     (4) Weight gain
     (5) Fever, chills, sweats
     (6) No enjoyment of life (anhedonia)
     (7) Pain
  b. Integument-related symptoms
     (1) Sores
     (2) Itching (pruritis)
     (3) Rash
     (4) Change in size or color of moles
     (5) Abnormal hair growth
     (6) Changes in nails
  c. Hematopoietic symptoms
     (1) Enlarged glands (lymphadenopathy)
     (2) Lumps anywhere
     (3) Urge to eat dirt (pica) or ice
     (4) Abnormal bleeding or excessive bruising
     (5) Frequent or unusual infections
  d. Endocrine symptoms
     (1) Heat intolerance
     (2) Cold intolerance
     (3) Decreased sexual drive
     (4) Salt craving
     (5) Enlarging glove and hat size
     (6) Excessive thirst (polydipsia)
  e. Musculoskeletal
     (1) Frequent fractures
     (2) Muscular weakness

      (3) Painful muscles
      (4) Joint pain and swelling
      (5) Low back pain
      (6) Paralysis
      (7) Movement difficulty
      (8) Pain in calf with walking (intermittent claudication)
      (9) Swollen leg
f. Eyes, ears, nose, and throat
      (1) Change in vision
      (2) Spots in visual field
      (3) Double vision (diplopia)
      (4) Loss of hearing
      (5) Ringing in the ears (tinnitus)
      (6) Drainage from nose
      (7) Decreased or altered sense of smell
      (8) Bloody nose (epistaxis)
      (9) Sore throat
     (10) Impaired speech
     (11) Painful tooth
     (12) Hoarseness
g. Head and neck
      (1) Headache
      (2) Dizzy (vertigo)
      (3) Light-headedness
      (4) Loss of consciousness (syncope)
      (5) Stiff neck
h. Breasts
      (1) Lump or mass
      (2) Discharge
      (3) Tenderness
i. Cardiovascular and pulmonary
      (1) Chest pain
      (2) Shortness of breath (dyspnea)
      (3) Shortness of breath when lying down and need to sit to breathe (orthopnea)
      (4) Wakening at night with dyspnea (paroxysmal nocturnal dyspnea)
      (5) Wheezing
      (6) Cough
      (7) Yellow or green sputum
      (8) Clear sputum

(9)   Bloody sputum (hemoptysis)
(10) Pounding sensation in chest (palpitations)
(11) (See Musculoskeletal and Integument for peripheral arterial and venous symptoms)
j. Gastrointestinal
(1)   (See **a.** General symptoms for appetite and weight changes)
(2)   Sticking sensation in throat (globus hystericus)
(3)   Difficulty swallowing (dysphagia)
(4)   Heartburn
(5)   Upper abdominal pain
(6)   Mid-lower abdominal pain
(7)   Nausea
(8)   Nonbloody vomiting (emesis)
(9)   Bloody emesis (hematemesis)
(10) Black stools (melena)
(11) Bloody stools (hematochezia)
(12) Difficult or infrequent bowel movements (constipation)
(13) Loose or frequent bowel movements (diarrhea)
(14) Yellow discoloration of sclerae and skin (jaundice)
(15) Dark urine like tea or a cola drink
(16) Excessive upper (belching or eructation) or lower (flatus) bowel gas
(17) Rectal pain (proctalgia), discharge, mass, hemorrhoid, or itching (pruritis ani)
(18) Lump in groin or scrotum
k. Urinary
(1)   Increased urinary frequency (polyuria)
(2)   Burning with urination (dysuria)
(3)   Getting up more than once during the night to void (nocturia)
(4)   Need to urinate suddenly and urgently (urgency)
(5)   Loss of urinary control (incontinence)
(6)   Bloody urine (hematuria)
(7)   Particulate matter in urine
(8)   Slow to get urinary stream started (hesitancy)
l. Genital, male
(1)   Urethral discharge
(2)   Penile sores or growths
(3)   Painful or swollen testicle
(4)   Impotence

      (5) Bloody ejaculation (hematospermia)
      (6) Retrograde ejaculation into bladder
      (7) Premature ejaculation
      (8) Decreased sexual drive
m. Genital, female
      (1) Vaginal discharge or itching
      (2) Sores or lumps
      (3) Painful menses (dysmenorrhea)
      (4) Absence of menses (amenorrhea)
      (5) Irregular, heavy menses (menometrorrhagia)
      (6) Hot flashes
      (7) Decreased sexual drive
      (8) Painful intercourse (dyspareunia)
      (9) Nonorgasmic
n. Neuropsychiatric
      (1) (See Head, Eyes, Ears, Nose, and Throat for cranial nerve symptoms)
      (2) (See Muscles for motor symptoms)
      (3) Numb, tingling sensation in extremities (paresthesia)
      (4) Decreased (hypesthesia) or absent (anesthesia) sensation
      (5) Tremor
      (6) Loss of balance
      (7) Staggering gait (ataxia)
      (8) Seizures
      (9) Bizarre, unrealistic thoughts (intrusive thoughts)
    (10) Bizarre, unrealistic perceptions (hallucinations)
    (11) Depression
    (12) Mania
    (13) Poor judgment, orientation, memory, attention, and concentration
    (14) Inability to get to sleep or stay asleep (insomnia)
    (15) Hypersomnolence
    (16) Nightmares
    (17) Anhedonia
    (18) Suicidal
    (19) Anxiety, nervousness
    (20) Symptoms without a disease explanation (somatization)
10. Physical examination[b]

11. Initial diagnostic formulations and treatment interventions (if any)[b]
12. Assessment: biopsychosocial description — **the patient's story**[c]
    a. Relationship story
       (1) Interviewer's responses
       (2) Patient's responses
       (3) Doctor-patient interaction
    b. Personal story
    c. Disease story/diagnosis
       (1) Biomedical
       (2) Psychiatric
13. Treatment and investigative plan[b]

[a]Many of these symptoms can occur in systems other than where listed.
[b]Not addressed in this book.
[c]Addressed in this book only to show the RPD designation.
Adapted from Morgan WL, Engel GL. *The Clinical Approach to the Patient.* Philadelphia: Saunders, 1969; and Billings AJ, Stoeckle JD. *The Clinical Encounter: A Guide to the Medical Interview and Case Presentation.* Chicago: Year Book, 1989.

As with most scientific endeavors, a well-organized, tightly knit written summary does not describe the discovery process itself. In fact, write-ups synthesize personal, primary, and secondary data from different parts of the interview. This synthesis is the write-up. The order in which data are discovered sometimes has little bearing on just where these data will be displayed in the written version.

Many use the following format (items 1 through 9), in the write-up for recording the history, physical examination, initial diagnostic formulations and treatment interventions, assessment, and treatment/investigative plans. All but the history are outside the scope of this book, but I include the others to illustrate the integration of the interview with the other four basic components of a formal patient evaluation. These components will be extensively addressed during clinical rotations.

Identifying Data
The student obtains identifying data (see pp. 181) from admitting records and other data that accompany the patient and by simple observation and inquiry.

Source and Reliability of Information

The source of data and its reliability reflect the quality of data obtained. The student should note any concerns; for example, "A translator was present but didn't seem to understand the patient very well and, in addition, the patient seemed embarrassed by the translator's presence. More information developed when the patient's husband, well-versed in English, arrived, and she was much more talkative."

Chief Complaint and Agenda

The chief complaint and patient's agenda clarify the patient's visit. Recalling that it may not have been presented first during the history, the chief complaint, or most bothersome symptom, serves as a powerful tool directing the focus of the written story. When possible, I advise citing the chief complaint in the patient's own words. Then a full agenda list should be summarized.

History of Present Illness (HPI)
and Other Current Active Problems (OCAP)

As noted on pp. 181–182, there are five specific aspects of the HPI (or OCAP): (1) an overview of pertinent symptoms (those that fit together to best describe the underlying disease process) and their time of onset, (2) specific symptom descriptors, (3) the absence of pertinent symptoms, (4) relevant secondary data, and (5) the personal context of these data. Through these five aspects of the history the student can convey a dynamic understanding of the patient's situation and thus prepare the reader to understand the full biopsychosocial description of the patient that is to be provided later (in assessment). For beginning clinical students, it can be helpful to put each category in a separate paragraph, as outlined below; as students gain experience, these categories can be condensed and interwoven.

Paragraph 1

An overview of all relevant symptoms, reflecting the chief complaint and other current problems, also identifies when each began. This information will most likely have arisen during the patient-centered process or during step 6 (getting an overview).

Paragraph 2

The student records all symptoms (primary data) relevant to the problem and expands upon each with a full recording of the seven descriptors (location, quality, quantitation, chronology and timing, setting, moderating factors, and associated symptoms). The descriptors can be recorded in this order, as shown for Mrs. Jones in Appendix B, and must be clearly anchored in the chronology and timing dimension. Rather than including all descriptors, experienced clinicians will often record only those of diagnostic significance. Students are advised, however, to remain comprehensive until their skills more fully develop. As students' skills and understanding of diseases increase, they will recognize more and more symptoms that belong in this paragraph; that is, the "associated symptom" category of the descriptors increases. Most data in this paragraph will have arisen in step 7 of the doctor-centered process.

Paragraph 3

The student next records the absence of pertinent symptoms. Thus, one would record the absence of symptoms from the same system of involvement as the chief complaint. As the student becomes more facile with hypothesis-testing and develops a better understanding of disease, the absence of other pertinent symptoms also is included. For example, in a patient with chest pain, the preclinical and beginning clinical student would record the absence of hemoptysis and dyspnea in this paragraph while the more advanced clinical student would also indicate the absence of joint pains and excessive sunburning if systemic lupus erythematosus was a diagnostic consideration (these are sometimes useful diagnostic symptoms). Data for this paragraph usually come from step 7 of the doctor-centered process.

Paragraph 4

Pertinent positive and negative nonsymptom (secondary) data are included in this paragraph. This includes data about, for example, doctors and health-care facilities, diagnostic tests and results, treatments and results, specific habits, occupation, and other nonsymptom data that are important to understanding the patient's problem—especially the etiology (cause) and pathogenesis (mechanism); for example, a history of smoking in someone with possible lung cancer, a recent coronary angiogram that was normal in a patient with chest pain, the use of birth control pills in patient with headaches; family history of sickle cell anemia in a boy with painful legs. These data will often have arisen in step 7 but also may have occurred in steps 8 to 12.

Paragraph 5

Although usually obtained first in the interview, mostly during the patient-centered process, personal data often are recorded last to enhance our understanding of how personal factors interact with the physical. The student explicitly links symptom, psychological, and emotional dimensions. It is in this final paragraph that the mind-body link is established. Although notable in Mrs. Jones' situation, we do not always find a clear causal relationship between personal factors and the disease problem. In all patients, however, we can describe a personal context of the physical problem.

The HPI, the most important part of the history, synthesizes the patient's personal and physical dimensions. Preclinical students, if called upon, simply record the chronology of primary data (including symptom descriptors), secondary data, and their personal dimensions. As one understands more about disease patterns later in training, one begins to record the patient's data in a way that leads another student or physician to the same diagnostic conclusion (given in assessment). The clinical student learns to selectively highlight portions of the story, still utilizing the five dimensions above, to provide data for and against the diagnosis she has made. Proceeding from a growing knowledge and skills base in clinical medicine, the student follows strict rules of clinical reasoning. Accordingly, data for and against the proposed diagnosis (hypothesis), and reasonable alternative diagnoses, are painstakingly and fairly recounted so another professional (often a preceptor) can make an informed decision. Mrs. Jones' HPI in Appendix B illustrates this diagnostic process.

The student includes only primary and secondary data in the HPI. Discussion and interpretation of the patient's problem come in the assessment. Interpretative comments can be made, however, when the clarity of data is in question; for example, "The patient alleges he underwent coronary bypass when hospitalized in 1983."

The OCAP is where the student records problems that are unrelated to the HPI but are nonetheless active and related to the patient's present health. Each of these areas requires a five-part approach similar to the HPI, although sometimes less extensive. Each usually has its own cardinal symptoms and its own physical and personal components.

Health Issues (HI)

All HI are recorded, as noted on pp. 182–183, and include ethical-social-spiritual issues, functional status, health-promoting and health-maintenance activities, and health hazards. When relevant, some of these already will have been recorded in the HPI or OCAP; for example, cigarette smoking habits are recorded in the HPI in most patients with shortness of breath and possible emphysema. Pertinent details, as outlined in Chapter 5, are provided in all areas; for example, dates, relevant people, when a Pap smear was last performed, number of cigarettes smoked daily and efforts to stop.

Past Medical History (PMH)
The PMH is recorded as noted on p. 183, often in the order suggested in the outline. It is detailed where necessary to provide understanding of the patient's health, but abbreviated for past events of little relevance to the patient's health. For example, in a patient admitted for a hernia repair, the student obtains extensive data about the patient's coronary artery bypass grafting 1 year earlier, not unlike what he would record in the HPI if the patient presented with chest pain. Although usually recorded in outline form, pertinent details are essential for all major problems; for example, symptoms, secondary data, dates, treatments, dosages of medications, types and outcome of adverse reactions to medications, and details of any complicated obstetric problem.

Social History (SH)
As outlined on pp. 183–184, the SH details the information, usually in narrative rather than tabular form. Only background and routine data are recorded in the SH. When details pertinent to current psychosocial issues have been elicited during the SH part of the interview, they are recorded in the HPI in the written record. Similarly, some SH data may have already been recorded, where relevant, as part of the OCAP or Identifying Data. Again, following Chapter 5 allows the student to record all relevant data.

Family History (FH)
The FH records information in the outline on pp. 184–185 in tabular form for the first two items and in a genogram for the third, as shown for Mrs. Jones in Appendix B. The tabular form is often more cumbersome and less informative than a genogram. Most important is to know who is available to the patient in a support role and who has or had, or fears they might have, anything like what the patient is suffering from. As noted before, some of these data may need to be included in the HPI/OCAP at times.

System Review of Items not Already Considered:
Review of Systems (ROS)

The ROS simply records system review symptoms not already considered during the HPI/OCAP or PMH. The beginning clinical level student often initially spends a lot of time here to get answers in still unaddressed systems, grouping the positives and negatives together in each system. This detail is necessary for learning purposes. More advanced students and graduates record only positive items, eventually noting only those that are significant.

Physical Examination

Physical examination findings, outside the province of this text, include, for example, notations of routine vital signs (temperature, pulse rate, respiratory rate, blood pressure, height, weight) and the details of examination in each system; for example, heart murmur heard on auscultation of the chest, an enlarged uterus on pelvic examination, or wax found on examining the ears.

Initial Diagnostic Formulations
and Treatment Interventions (if any)

Also outside the scope of this text, initial interventions by the student or others, which occur largely in acute situations, are recorded here; for example, a blood count in someone who is bleeding, an electrocardiogram in someone with chest pain, administration of adrenalin to a patient with an acute allergic reaction, or an x-ray of the abdomen in a patient injured in a traffic accident. These data should not be confused with secondary data obtained before the patient came under the student's care, which are already recorded in the HPI or PMH.

Assessment: Biopsychosocial Description —
The Patient's Story

Also outside the scope of an interviewing textbook, except to illustrate the RPD designation, the assessment is where the student gives the complete RPD description and discusses how data were interpreted to arrive at this. Sometimes, however, additional observation or diagnostic investigation is required before a full biopsychosocial description can be made. In the disease category, when descriptions are definitive enough to allow identification of a disease, the disease itself is recorded. When descriptions are not sufficient to permit a disease diagnosis, a succinct and pertinent description of the problem is recorded and called a "problem" to contrast it to a diagnosis.

At whatever level of resolution, the biopsychosocial description is recorded using the RPD components (see highlights) as illustrated in the following example:

Relationship story
  Interviewer's responses: liked patient, but difficult to talk about possible appendectomy for fear of making patient feel worse about job and home situation [*Note how this links all three RPD components*]
  Patient's personality: a few dependent features within the range of normal
  Interaction: cordial, cooperative, "same wavelength"
Personal story: worried about losing job because of illness and about increased demand on sick spouse. Is in a new job and does not want to become unemployed again.
Disease story (diagnoses/problems)
  Biomedical
  1. Abdominal pain of 48 hours duration with recent localization to right lower quadrant, accompanied by absent bowel sounds, involuntary guarding, and rebound tenderness [*This is a "problem" description because a diagnosis was not yet possible. Full discussion of how the interviewer arrived at the interpretation often is included here.*]
  2. Degenerative arthritis of knees and hands [*A diagnosis*]
  3. Type II (adult-onset) diabetes mellitus [*A diagnosis*]
  Psychiatric: past history of depression

Treatment and Investigative Plan
Also outside the province of this text, treatment and investigative plans follow logically from the above assessment and could include, for example, a blood count, an X-ray of the abdomen, and exploratory surgery for likely appendicitis.

Presenting the Patient's Story

Students and graduates frequently tell patients' stories to other professionals. These verbal presentations are valuable for learning and teaching, and they are the medium for communication among professionals. Although presentations are difficult at the outset, beginning clinical level students must quickly master them. They demonstrate the interviewer's ability to elicit and synthesize large amounts of data, her skills in communicating with others, and the way she sees the patient as a person.

There are three types of presentation: very brief, standard, and prolonged. Very brief presentations last no more than a minute or so and orient a surrogate to key problems in nonurgent situations; for example, "I'll be in the clinic all afternoon. Mr. Johnson in Room 345 has pneumonia but is doing okay on penicillin. Check his blood cultures when they're out at four o'clock P.M. His wife should be in about then too; let her know all is okay and I'll be back to talk with her around suppertime. Thanks."

The standard, 3 to 10 minute presentation conveys full, pertinent information to a listener unfamiliar with the patient. Such presentations are useful teaching exercises as well as being relied on to transmit critical information to other caretakers. Students and residents make these presentations to preceptors or senior residents at morning reports, on rounds, and in the clinic. The new clinical student synthesizes personal, primary, and secondary data into a logical diagnosis, and then presents it cogently and interestingly. Presentations follow the same format as the write-up, including the logic of clinical reasoning, but are much more condensed and contain only the most essential data.

The following is an example of a standard presentation—using Mrs. Jones as our subject. (This is a transcript of the junior student's presentation of Mrs. Jones' initial evaluation to his preceptor in the clinic. Although some preceptors may want more detail, most prefer a succinct, pertinent presentation.)

Identifying Data, Source and Reliability of Data, Chief Complaint, and Other Major Agenda Items

The student gives these in one or two sentences, and conveys the broad strokes of the situation.

> *Joanne Jones is a 38-year-old married white woman who is a lawyer, a reliable historian, and self-referred for headaches of 3 months duration and to get established with a primary care doctor. She also is concerned about stress at work, a past history of ulcerative colitis, and a recent cold.*

History of the Present Illness (HPI)
If we can organize the HPI chronologically, the listener will better

understand the subsequent diagnosis or problem identification we came to. This doesn't mean that a preceptor will agree with the analysis, but it allows her to judge the data and rationale the student used. One avoids bias and emphasizes pros and cons of diagnostic data. To continue with Mrs. Jones' presentation, we hear the following:

Throbbing, nonradiating right temporal headaches associated with nausea and photophobia began suddenly 3 months ago. These have progressively worsened, especially in the last month, so that they now occur 2 to 3 times weekly and last 2 to 12 hours, during which time they progressively increase in severity. They are quite severe (worse than having a baby) and make her miss work. An ice bag and dark room seem to help some.

She has been well between headaches and there are no other symptoms, particularly scintillating scotomata or those suggesting neurological disease, meningitis, or head injury. I get no history of arthritis or anything suggesting a collagen disease.

An aunt likely had migraine and the patient has used birth control pills for 6 years. She had to go to the Emergency Department once a week ago, receiving a narcotic injection, and only a blood and urine study were done and we don't have these results yet.

Headaches clearly relate to anger at her boss, who criticizes and disdains her often, and they don't occur when he's not around. She is gradually replacing him as the lead attorney in GHI Corporation, and he is resisting this more than her Board had said he would. She's mad at them too. She also had headaches as a child when her mother criticized her unfairly and repeatedly. Talking about these problems brought on the headache during our interview. Although her support system is fairly good, she's getting worse and, if there's no help with this, she may quit her job. She's not depressed and has had no similar problems getting along in the past.

Notice that the student has covered the five components of the HPI we discussed as part of the write-up. The student next reports only pertinent OCAP, HI, PMH, SH, FH, and ROS data.

Except for chronic stress on the job and being 'workaholic,' she takes good care of herself from a health maintenance standpoint: seat belts, good aerobics almost daily, low-fat and low-salt diet, no addicting substances, and no risky habits. She has been followed regularly, including Pap smears.

Her past history is significant for what was diagnosed as mild ulcerative colitis in 1982 when she was hospitalized at the University Hospital in her home town. She'd had bloody diarrhea off and on for 3 months then and responded to 3 months of prednisone and about a year of sulfasalazine after her work-up was completed. It sounds like both sigmoidoscopy and barium enema were done as well as several other tests and I'm sending for the records. She was followed regularly by a Dr. Jergens and was asymptomatic until November 1991 when nonbloody diarrhea occurred and sigmoidoscopy and barium enema showed minimal changes in what she calls the "distal sigmoid colon." No surgery has ever been advised and she continues without symptoms, having responded almost immediately to another course of sulfasalazine which she took for 6 months. A sigmoidoscopy 6 months ago was said to be normal.

Except for two uncomplicated obstetric confinements, a mild but now cleared respiratory infection recently, and her only urinary tract infection 8 months ago, she has been in good health.

Aspirin, 6 to 8 daily, is the only other medication. There are no drug sensitivities or allergies.

The SH is significant only in that this job was a big step forward professionally. The FH is not further contributory. ROS reveals nothing more.

Physical Examination

Only pertinent data are given, both normal and abnormal, focusing at the outset on a vivid general description of the patient and relevant vital signs. (Because physical examination is outside the province of this text, only a brief report of the exam is presented; most preceptors would prefer that it be more complete and specific.)

Physical examination shows a normotensive healthy appearing woman who is attractive, friendly, and shows no mental status abnormalities. Head and neck are normal and without bruises or tenderness. Detailed neurological evaluation shows no abnormalites of cranial nerves, reflexes, cerebellar function, extrapyramidal function, or motor/sensory function. She does have a midsystolic click along the left sternal border but there is no murmur or other abnormality.

Initial Diagnostic and Treatment Interventions (if any)

As in the write-up, these usually emergency actions have been obtained under the student's and his team's direction.

No diagnostic or treatment interventions have been made and we do not yet have the lab data from a week ago.

Assessment: Biopsychosocial Description — The Patient's Story

Assessment is equally cogent, as shown in Mrs. Jones' story.

(1) We got along well and she indicated liking my approach. I liked her but I think I cut the conversation short when she was talking about some sexual problems she had. I didn't know what to say. (2) Mrs. Jones is under severe

stress from the conflict with her boss on a new job. (3) In turn, this has precipitated migraine headaches, with a typical clinical picture of intermittent throbbing and photophobia and a family history. The birth control pills could be a factor as well. Less likely is a stress tension headache: I wouldn't expect this to be so intermittent, severe, or throbbing. Meningitis, subdural hematoma, and a vasculitis all are extremely unlikely. She has ulcerative colitis, the recent cold, a urinary tract infection last summer, and probably mitral valve prolapse that is not symptomatic.

Treatment and Investigative Plan

This is equally brief and to the point, as shown with Mrs. Jones. In complicated cases, this and the assessment are much more extensive.

For the headaches, I'd suggest we start her on ergotamine tartrate with caffeine tablets for the acute headaches. Prophylactic treatment, with a beta blocker or calcium channel blocker, may be necessary but I'd like to see first what our other measures do. Likewise, if she doesn't do better, we may need to stop the birth control pills. We've already discussed strategies for working with her boss and I'd like to follow up in about a week to see how this is progressing and perhaps develop some new strategies. I think she'd also benefit from knowing a relaxation procedure that I can show her. I don't think any laboratory investigation is needed now but, should she not respond, we might want to reconsider. We'll get records from the Emergency Department and from Dr. Jergens, and I think she needs a follow-up sigmoidoscopy sometime soon. A return appointment for 1 week is okay with her.

As noted, the student included the five components of the written HPI: chronological overview of the story, the dimensions of each symptom, pertinent positives and negatives, course of the problem and relevant secondary data, and the personal contextual aspects. In the assessment, all RPD components are included so that the listener obtains the full, integrated biopsychosocial description.

Longer presentations more closely resemble the written report. These usually are for presenting an interesting patient problem for teaching purposes (10–15 minutes), or for evaluating students' grasp of their patients (30–45 minutes). The time available determines how much is included. The student allows relatively more time for the assessment and its discussion, either to pose the problem for discussion or to show her understanding of the patient.

Not only does the student investigate and formulate the problem beforehand but, once the presentation is outlined, it can be practiced; audiotaping and feedback from other students can be especially helpful. Notes are best kept to a minimum and brief presentations go best with no notes used at all. Longer presentations usually require notes, which are not read but referred to for organizational purposes. Concluding summaries are often helpful in longer presentations.

References

1. Barrows HS, Pickell GC. *Developing Clinical Problem-Solving Skills—A Guide to More Effective Diagnosis and Treatment.* New York: Norton Medical Books, 1991.
2. Tresolini CP, Pew-Fetzer Task Force. *Health Professions Education and Relationship-Centered Care.* San Francisco: Pew Health Professions Commission, 1994.
3. American Psychiatric Association. *Diagnostic and Statistical Manual of Mental Disorders* (4th ed.). Washington, DC: American Psychiatric Association, 1994.
4. Smith RC, Hoppe RB. The patient's story: integrating the patient- and physician-centered approaches to interviewing. *Ann Intern Med* 115:470–477, 1991.
5. Regier D, Goldberg I, Taube C. The de facto mental health services system. *Arch Gen Psychiatry* 35:685–693, 1978.
6. Kessler, LG, Burns BJ, Shapiro S, et al. Psychiatric diagnoses of medical service users: evidence from the epidemiologic catchment area program. *Am J Pub Health* 77:18–24, 1987.
7. Frankel RM, Beckman HB. Effective interviewing and intervention for alcohol problems. In Lipkin M, Putnam SM, Lazare A (eds.), *The Medical Interview.* New York: Springer-Verlag, 1995. Pp. 511–524.
8. Mitchell WJT (ed). *On Narrative.* Chicago: University of Chicago Press, 1981.
9. Kerby AP. *Narrative and the Self.* Bloomington, IN: Indiana University Press, 1991.
10. Bohm D. *Wholeness and the Implicate Order.* London: Routledge and Kegan Paul, 1980.
11. Anderson H, Goolishian HA. Human systems as linguistic systems: Preliminary and evolving ideas about the implications for clinical theory. *Family Process* 27:371–393, 1988.

Patient Education

Patient education often is overlooked in medical communication textbooks. Educating patients means giving them information and, where necessary, motivating them to act on it. To this point we have addressed only gathering information from the patient and establishing a relationship. As soon as the database permits, however, educating the patient becomes equally important. Only a small percentage of interactions leads to mechanical, doctor-given treatments, such as an injection or a manipulation. Most treatment is in the form of instructions to patients who will, themselves, carry out the treatment. Our patients take their pills, go for x-rays and tests, and keep their appointments. We do not do it for them. Therefore, educating the patient is a key element in therapeutics [1–4].

Although patient education occurs throughout the entire encounter, we usually emphasize that function toward the end of an interaction. Consider these patients. The first, new to our care and similar to Mrs. Jones, requires information on the student's present findings, answers to questions, and diagnostic and treatment plans for the future. The second is a follow-up visit by a patient who wants to resume an exercise program after recovering from a badly sprained ankle. This request was made when the student was using the patient-centered process. The student devotes a large part of the interaction, following the doctor-centered process and physical examination, to explaining an exercise program. The third patient asks for no information but the doctor wants to discuss a topic that the patient does not ask about. The doctor first listens to the patient's needs using the patient-centered process and attends to necessary details using the doctor-centered process. Having learned during this or previous visits that the patient smokes cigarettes the doctor also wants to discuss the need to stop smoking. Education thus involves items stemming from either patient- or physician-centered concerns.

Education occurs in two categories. (1) Sometimes the interviewer needs to provide information, whether good or bad news, but is not challenged with the task of motivating the patient to act on it; for example, the patient above is informed about an improving ankle and the exercise program requested. (2) Often the interviewer has to give information and to motivate the patient to act on it; for example, the patient may not be ready to agree to a cigarette cessation program. The interviewer must then enlist the patient as an active decision maker and partner in therapy [2,5–7]. Such negotiation may be implicit and easily agreed upon. Often, though, the interviewer must explicitly negotiate with the patient about the patient's and doctor's behaviors and roles, as with the cigarette smoker.

The interviewer needs patient-centered skills not yet addressed to educate patients effectively. As might be expected, understanding the personal context of the educational issue and developing a healthy relationship remain essential [8].

Providing Information

Giving Routine Data

Much of our informing seems simple; for example, prescribing treatment and diagnostic tests, giving results of tests, and explaining causes of problems. But many patients do not understand information provided in spoken or written form and, still worse, forget 40 percent of it [9]. Equally problematic, most doctors underestimate their patients' desire for information, especially that of shy or inarticulate patients, and spend very little time informing patients [10].

The following eight steps, outlined in Table 9-1, greatly enhance patient understanding and memory [11,12].

1. Determine the patient's present understanding. For example, students often have to ask, "Before I start explaining things, let me check first and see what you already know about heart tests."
2. Give the most important instructions and advice before other information and stress their top priority; e.g., "I'm going to start with what is most important for your health, so this is what you most need to remember." This will enhance the likelihood of recall and compliance with the most important message.
3. Categorize data where possible; e.g., "First let's talk about your heart medicines and then. . . ."

Table 9-1.   Providing information

1. Check baseline understanding
2. Give instructions first—and stress their importance
3. Categorize information
4. Make clear, simple, and short statements about one major bit of information at a time
5. Advice should concern specific patient behaviors
6. Encourage questions
7. Check understanding
8. Repeat the message; write it down if necessary

Adapted from Ley P, et al. Improving doctor-patient communication in general practice. *J R Coll Gen Pract* 26:720–724, 1976.
Ley P. Memory for medical information. *Br J Soc Clin Psychol* 18:245–255, 1979.

4. Make a clear, short statement with simple words about one bit of data at a time.
5. Recommend specific behaviors the patient is to perform; e.g., "In the mornings, walk around the block for 15 minutes, sit and rest for 15 minutes, and then repeat this once more. Do the same in the evenings."
6. Encourage patients to ask questions.
7. Ask questions to check the patient's understanding of major points. Do not provide more data until the initial material is clarified and assimilated.
8. Repeat the most important messages, and be prepared to write the information down if necessary; be sure the patient can read the writing and understand the words.

Giving Bad News
Sometimes we have bad news for our patients. We can expect them to find such news very hard to hear; for example, a diagnosis of cancer or AIDS. In addition to a patient-centered attitude and a supportive approach, the following guidelines, summarized in Table 9-2 [13], are useful.

Plan Ahead
The interviewer ensures that data are complete and accurate, that she fully understands them, and that she knows how to proceed. Patients will almost certainly ask questions about diagnosis, prognosis, and subsequent treatment. The interviewer also prepares by considering her own grief and loss. Failure to attend to one's own responses often leads to their unplanned, deleterious intrusion

Table 9-2. Giving bad news*

1. Plan ahead
   a. Be sure information is complete and well understood
   b. Attend to one's own reactions
   c. Have necessary others present
   d. Rehearse in light of patient's personality and other unique features
2. Personally arrange the meeting, be sure enough time is available, and avoid use of intermediaries or a telephone
3. Ensure a safe, comfortable setting
4. Determine patient's readiness to hear the information and his level of understanding of the situation
5. Give the bad news clearly and succinctly
   a. Give only one bit at a time
   b. Encourage questions and answer directly — clearly correct misperceptions or overreactions
   c. Encourage emotional expression
   d. Do not falsely reassure but always convey hope, even if just the interviewer's support
   e. Be comfortable with silence and do not rush the patient
   f. Accept that you may be able to do nothing but be there with the patient
   g. Encourage follow-up questions and check patient's understanding
   h. Provide necessary additional information, repeating the above process until sufficient information has been given or the patient's tolerance reached
   i. Explore impact on patient's life and her beliefs about the implications of the bad news
   j. Determine if patient is suicidal — and make necessary immediate arrangements if so
6. Develop a plan
   a. Ensure a support system
   b. Inform others
   c. Explicitly schedule follow-up visits or telephone calls — give home telephone number
   d. Initiate follow-up if patient does not
   e. Discuss appropriate diagnostic and treatment considerations

*Emotion-seeking and emotion-handling skills are used throughout.
Adapted from Quill TE, Townsend P. Bad news: delivery, dialogue, and dilemmas. Arch Intern Med 1991;151:463–468.

into the patient's situation; for example, a doctor provides a falsely reassuring picture because of his own unrecognized loss in learning that a well-liked patient has widespread metastatic cancer. One determines who else, if anyone, needs to be informed and if this person should be at the initial meeting. When the patient is young or of limited competence, a responsible person must be present. Similarly, a psychologically fragile or denying patient needs a responsible and supportive person. If such a supportive person is available, many of us, strong or weak, benefit from that presence. On the other hand, the patient may not want anyone present, and the interviewer accepts this initially. When bad news can be anticipated, one arranges a follow-up meeting and negotiates in advance who will be there.

Rarely, giving bad news might be medically or psychologically dangerous; for example, the interviewer has additional bad news for a patient having an acute heart attack or a patient who is suicidal. Even here, I advise against long delays. Sometimes families ask that information be withheld from the patient, often to "protect" them. The interviewer may accommodate this briefly, for example, to bring a close relative home, but a delay should not be prolonged. Patients have the right to information about themselves.

Prior to the difficult discussion, the student should jot down important points she plans to make. One can even rehearse the key statements aloud. Sometimes that makes for a more coherent message and a more sensitive interaction. It helps to incorporate information about the patient's personality style, spiritual life, beliefs, and support system in one's preparation.

Personally Arrange a Meeting with the Patient

If advance arrangements have not been made, the student personally makes them but avoids giving the bad news on the phone; for example, "Some of your lab tests are back. They're too complicated to talk about on the phone, so I'd like you and your wife to come in later today so we can discuss them." This sort of "message framing" sounds innocuous but will probably worry the patient, so one tries to arrange the meeting as soon as possible and provide sufficient time.

Ensure a Safe and Comfortable Setting

A private office or room suffices. Avoid discussions in hallways, coffee shops, or any other place where privacy and comfort are unlikely. The interviewer establishes an atmosphere of warmth and safety by nonverbal means (e.g., shake hands), undivided and unhurried attention, ensuring the patient's physical comfort, and by arranging the situation so that no interruptions occur.

Determine the Patient's Readiness to Listen and Understanding of the Situation

The interviewer tries to learn how ready and able the patient is to hear the bad news; this involves learning about whatever else might be going on in the patient's life at the time that might be more important and more stressful [8]. If the patient is not ready, the interviewer must help by allowing the patient to control the pace and flow of information. This includes addressing issues perceived as needing disposition (e.g., answering a business call) or more pressing (e.g., being certain the baby-sitter knows where the patient is) and, then, gently asking if the patient is ready to proceed and address a serious health matter. Interviewers look for emotional content and, in doing so, may discover fear of anticipated bad news or exaggerated anxiety about its implications. Rarely, the patient really may not want to hear the news. We have to consider this option and in such cases try to inform other responsible parties.

The interviewer next determines the patient's understanding of the problem. This includes her knowledge about the diagnosis and her beliefs about its implication for prognosis and treatment. The interviewer establishes these data with focused, open-ended questions such as, "Tell me first about your understanding of the situation and what concerns you have."

Give the Bad News

The interviewer prefaces the bad news by indicating that a problem exists; for example, "I'm afraid I have some difficult news to give you." This lessens the shock of the bad news and allows the patient to brace himself for what is to come. The interviewer then gives a clear, direct, and brief message. Only one bit of the most important information is given at a time; for example, "Your mammogram is very indicative of cancer." A common understanding of terms, such as cancer, cannot be assumed and may need clarification.

The interviewer follows the patient's lead in deciding how far and how fast to proceed, accepting questions and listening for emotions. The interviewer gives clear answers and explanations and clarifies any misperceptions or overreactions; for example, "Yes, surgery will be needed but they usually don't remove the entire breast any more." If emotion is not forthcoming, the interviewer uses emotion-seeking skills. The interaction will evolve as the patient expresses emotion and a desire for more information. The interviewer must tread a fine line. We do not want the patient to feel pushed or overwhelmed. Nor do we want to leave the patient isolated with her fear, anger, or grief. Gentle emotion-seeking and emotion-handling usually works best.

The interviewer avoids false reassurance but still conveys hope; for example, to a newly diagnosed AIDS patient, "I know it looks bad but treatment is working better all the time, and there's a lot of research going on." Sometimes, though, the interviewer himself provides the only immediate hope. The student makes his presence and support explicit and conveys appropriate nonverbal support (arm around shoulder, holding hand), often the first link in eventually restoring meaning and hope. The interviewer reassures the patient that he will not be abandoned—a common and weighty fear. Silence and a quiet presence are powerful. One's own genuine emotions are appropriate and often consoling [14]. Alleviation of suffering can be most successful when the interviewer abandons efforts at reassurance and recognizes there may be nothing to do but be available and provide support. The student will be most effective if he can establish and develop this relationship over many encounters, as might occur in a primary care setting [14]. The first visit is just the beginning.

After the initial shock passes, the interviewer encourages questions and checks the patient's understanding. In tension-laden situations many people do not assimilate information well and can develop an erroneous understanding, often one that is worse than the actual situation. For example, when informed of cancer or AIDS, many expect to die within a few months. To offset this, it can help to tape-record the interaction and give the tape to the patient [14].

As additional information is exchanged, further feelings may be displayed and the interviewer again addresses these using emotion-seeking skills and the NURS tetrad (see Chap. 2). As the interaction evolves, the interviewer reinforces the patient's other supports, her strengths, and her prior abilities in dealing with adversity. The interviewer needs to learn the impact of the bad news on the patient's life and on the lives of others. The interviewer also gauges how well the patient is handling the information and tries not to overwhelm her. Additional meetings often are necessary to allow sufficient assimilation of all information. The interviewer also must determine if the patient is suicidal. This can be done only by direct inquiry; for example, "This is a lot to throw at you and I know you're quite down. Do thoughts of hurting yourself arise, you know, taking your life?". While the student will learn about the suicidal patient in psychiatry rotations, if suicidal intent is detected, she needs to hear more about it and often asks for immediate outside help.

Develop a Plan

Ensure satisfactory support. This includes medical and psychological professionals as well as family, friends, church, support groups, and others. With some patients, the interviewer may need to assist in obtaining support, either because there is little of it or the patient is too defeated to seek it out.

If the student plans to inform significant others, she negotiates specific plans with the patient beforehand. Usually this presents no problem; the patient wants certain others informed or will inform them on her own. On other occasions, though, the student must discuss with the patient any plans to exclude other concerned members of the family. They may need to be informed for medical, legal, and humanistic reasons.

The interviewer schedules a follow-up visit in the very near future and may make a follow-up telephone call later the same day. The interviewer might give the patient his home phone number and would initiate follow-up actions if the patient fails to make a scheduled visit or call.

The student initiates psychological or medical interventions. A sedative or brief course of an anxiolytic can be beneficial. Prescribing specific tasks helps the overwhelmed patient; for example, who and how to tell the news, writing down questions, and talking to others with similar problems. Also, the interviewer arranges additional diagnostic and therapeutic interventions; for example, referral to a surgeon.

Providing Information and Motivating Patients to Act on It

The same principles obtain when patients require motivation. In addition, though, the interviewer now tries to persuade the patient to accept a course not previously chosen. Focusing upon the doctor's agenda to correct an adverse health habit, such as smoking cigarettes, may lead to a conflicted interview. While the interviewer encourages her agenda, such an action requires skillful negotiation to establish the patient as responsible and in charge.

We now consider the three aspects of educating a patient to change behaviors: (1) informing and motivating, (2) obtaining a commitment, and (3) negotiating a specific plan. When no commitment is obtained, the interviewer works to maintain the relationship and keep the door open for other problems as well as for later educational activities.

We can assume that we are working with emotionally charged material. The interviewer uses emotion-seeking and emotion-handling skills throughout, particularly at points of resistance. The student needs a sound clinical base to effectively educate the patient. Because the specific approach to each adverse health habit is unique and varied, I present only a general guide. As students learn clinical medicine, they can easily fit specific clinical information into the template outlined in Table 9-3 [1].

Establish an Information Base and Motivate the Patient

As always, the interviewer begins by determining the patient's knowledge base and readiness to change; for example, "What do you know about the health impact of cigarette smoking? Where are you in thinking about quitting?" Following this, the interviewer informs the patient, if needed, about the adverse potential of his present actions (smoking cigarettes, alcohol or drug use, lack of exercise, being overweight, stressful life, not using condoms). For example, a patient who was not aware of an adverse impact might be informed that smoking cigarettes is associated with a 10 percent risk of developing lung cancer, a greater chance of developing bronchitis and emphysema, even more risk for developing cardiovascular disease (heart attack, stroke), and a general reduction of 6 to 7 years in life expectancy.

Next, the student makes a brief, explicit recommendation; for example, "For health purposes, you need to quit smoking completely." The student follows with a statement that improved health and other benefits (cost, odor) will follow; for example, "By quitting cigarettes your health improves immediately and after being off them a year, the risk for heart attacks and strokes is almost as though you'd never smoked."

The student also incorporates awareness of the patient's personality style to increase motivation. For example, specific discussion of the literature would enhance acceptance with an obsessive-

Table 9-3. Informing and motivating*

1. Establish an information base and motivate the patient
   a. Determine knowledge base and readiness for change
   b. Clearly inform about adverse potential of health habit needing change
   c. Make brief, explicit recommendation for change
   d. Motivate patient
      (1) Informing of health and other benefits from change
      (2) Using knowledge of personality
      (3) Highlighting patient's capacity for change
      (4) Emphasizing that help is available
      (5) Indicating that past failures do not bode poorly
   e. Check understanding and desire for change
2. Obtain a commitment
   a. Reinforce commitment
   b. Set expectations for success
   c. Reaffirm commitment
   d. Manage a decision against advice
3. Negotiate a specific plan
   a. Start with detailed understanding of role in the patient's life of habit to be changed
   b. Involve patient actively in plan, including when to begin and the specific details of its implementation
   c. Include medical interventions where applicable
   d. Check understanding and reaffirm plan
   e. Set follow-up

*Emotion-seeking and emotion-handling skills are used throughout.
Adapted from Stoffelmayr B, Hoppe RB, Weber N. Facilitating patient participation: The doctor-patient encounter. *Primary Care* 16:265–278, 1989.

compulsive patient, indicating the potential adverse effect on one's appearance would appeal to a histrionic person, and an appeal that complications of smoking could prevent her continued care of a spouse would be compelling to a patient with a self-defeating style.

The interviewer also persuades by emphasizing the patient's interests the habit could interfere with (e.g., see grandchildren grow up) and his capabilities for change; for example, "You've really done a lot at the church and are known as a doer. You could add this to your list of achievements, set a good example for many, and gain the benefit of saving a lot of money." Gauging from the patient's style and response to suggested interventions, the interviewer, variously, may need to be a cheerleader, politician, diplomat, confidant, and disciplinarian. The interviewer should communicate in the way the patient best understands. On the other hand, the more the interviewer pressures the patient to change her behavior, the more likely she is to resist. The patient must lead. When the interviewer finds out what she wants to do, then he can offer appropriate help.

The interviewer can say that help is available and effective; for example, "I'll be working with you weekly on this if you decide to go ahead, and there are smokers' groups and medications that are helpful as well. We've had some great results." This offsets the pessimistic view that nothing can be done. To further encourage the patient, the interviewer can tell the patient that having failed before at changing a bad habit bodes well for future efforts because most successful patients have had many unsuccessful previous attempts.

The interviewer repeatedly intersperses emotion-seeking ("how're you doing with this; it's a lot to ask of you") and emotion-handling skills ("it has been difficult for you to quit, I know, and I understand what it's like. I'm impressed that you're considering that we might work together on it"). These skills are more effective with recalcitrant patients than is repeated education or encouragement efforts. We need to understand the patient more and convey this to him. Usually, he already understands us. Still, we check the patient's understanding, particularly the recommendation being made; for example, "We've talked about a lot of stuff and I want to be sure I haven't confused the issue. What do you hear me telling you?"

Obtain a Commitment

Trying to obtain a commitment may be the most awkward part of the interaction, and tension can lead the interviewer to be vague, indirect, or to provide a loophole for escape. The interviewer might say, "We need to decide now if you want to make a commitment to working on this." The student must allow the silence and awkwardness that often follows such a statement. Patients are indeed on the spot and need to wrestle with the issue. They may have little experience in making such decisions for themselves, but the decision must be theirs.

If the patient does commit to a change, the student should support such a plan and reaffirm his availability and that of other help. In addition, the interviewer sets expectations of success and reinforces the patient for making a change; for example, "I'm impressed that you're willing to work on such a big change. I know it will be a stretch but I think you can do it."

Before moving to the next stage, the student will once again check and ask the patient to affirm her decision. For example, one might say, "To be sure we're clear, could you repeat what you want to do?"

Negotiate a Specific Plan

The student needs to understand the details of the behavior to be changed so that an effective plan can be agreed upon. In our example of cigarette smoking, the interviewer wants the details of when the patient smokes, the most important times for smoking (e.g., while drinking coffee), what stresses prompt smoking (e.g., work), and what situations might make the patient resume smoking once stopped (e.g., "having a beer with the boys"). Strategies for change must address these issues and, at the same time, be compatible with the patient's daily life.

As usual, the interviewer involves the patient actively in identifying problem areas and solutions. For example, a cigarette smoker first identified drinking beer with his friends as a difficult time, and the interviewer then facilitated the patient's decision not to join these friends at the tavern for the first month or so. Similarly, the patient decided to tell them and others that he was quitting smoking. (Some patients will not want to let others know.) The patient agreed to stop smoking over an upcoming holiday when he would be away from his smoking friends and the stress at work. (Some prefer to quit while they can stay busy.) The patient decided to drink herbal tea instead of coffee and to chew gum to replace the cigarettes. Whatever the patient's plan, an interviewer who facilitates the patient's active involvement achieves the greatest success. Only the patient can find those solutions that are unique to his life circumstance.

With some habits, the interviewer encourages a "step at a time" approach. For example, while smoking requires complete abstinence, a diet often works best when just a few foods are decreased. In initiating a low-cholesterol diet, the interviewer negotiates decisions about which foods to reduce (e.g., eggs), the amount of reduction (e.g., one instead of three), and the meal from which they are reduced (e.g., breakfast). Only if the cholesterol does not fall would further negotiation be required (e.g., stop the remaining egg at breakfast, substitute margarine for butter, and reduce red meat intake to twice weekly).

When applicable, the student negotiates medical interventions as well. For example, medications for elevated cholesterol are seldom used until stringent dietary measures have been shown ineffective.

On the other hand, nicotine-replacement regimens (gums, patches) are sometimes used initially if the patient wants this help to stop smoking. Similarly, some patients might want to participate in group work for support from the ongoing efforts of others. Some patients, however, want no medications, no group work, or no other medical interventions and prefer to "do it on my own."

After negotiating a plan, the student asks the patient to repeat the specific plan to be implemented. This reinforces it and allows any misunderstanding to be clarified. Agreement on the timetable is especially important. Before ending the interaction, the interviewer also reinforces and supports the patient's commitment and sets follow-up plans. It is sometimes necessary to write this out for the patient to take home.

When a Commitment Is Not Obtained

A negotiated approach allows and accommodates the option that the patient may discard the interviewer's advice. The interviewer non-judgmentally inquires about refusal, being careful that the patient does not feel pressured, and clarifies any misunderstanding.

When the patient rejects a recommendation, the interviewer can ask, "What would it take to make you change your mind?" [15]. Our cigarette smoker, for example, might answer with, "Well, a heart attack or cancer, I guess." The answer itself sometimes helps the patient realize how really dangerous the habit is and that now is the time to act.

The interviewer makes explicit that, while she may disagree, she does accept the patient's decision. Students should defuse differences or tension that might interfere with subsequent care. The interviewer reassures the patient that he will not pressure or abandon the patient—but that he will continue to gently explore the patient's readiness to change. One empathic technique is to express understanding of the patient's dilemma; for example, "I can see you are caught in a bind. On the one hand, you're tired of these chest colds and want to stop smoking. On the other hand, you enjoy smoking and find it releases stress at work. So you both want to quit and want not to. That's a real squeeze!"

Summary

Treating and educating the patient involve both patient-centered and doctor-centered processes. The interviewer checks the patient's readiness for the information, establishes a baseline of the patient's understanding and desires, informs her to the extent necessary, determines his commitment to action where needed, and negotiates specific plans. Sometimes, especially with adverse health habits, the interviewer also must try to motivate the patient to act upon the information provided. The interviewer frequently checks the patient's comprehension and always reaffirms plans. The more difficult the situation, the more the interviewer uses emotion-seeking and emotion-handling skills.

References

1. Stoffelmayr B, Hoppe RB, Weber N. Facilitating patient participation: The doctor-patient encounter. *Primary Care* 16:265–278, 1989.
2. Grueninger UJ, Duffy FD, Goldstein MG. Patient Education in the Medical Encounter: How to Facilitate Learning, Behavior, Change, and Coping. In Lipkin M, Putnam SM, Lazare A (eds.), *The Medical Interview*. New York: Springer-Verlag, 1995. Pp. 122–133.
3. Grueninger UJ, Goldstein MG, Duffy DF. Patient education in hypertension: Five essential steps. *Hypertension* 7 (suppl 3): s93–s98, 1989.
4. Prochaska JO, DiClemente CC. Towards a Comprehensive Model of Change. In Miller WR, Heather N (eds.), *Treating Addictive Behaviors: Processes of Change*. New York: Plenum Press, 1986. Pp. 3–27.
5. Lazare A, et al. Studies on a Negotiated Approach to Patienthood. In Stoeckle JD (ed.), *Encounters Between Patients and Doctors*. Cambridge: The MIT Press, 1987. Pp. 413–432.
6. Lazare A, Eisenthal S, Wasserman L. The customer approach to patienthood: attending to patient requests in a walk-in clinic. *Arch Gen Psychiatry* 32:552–558, 1975.
7. Quill TE. Partnerships in patient care: a contractual approach. *Ann Intern Med* 98:228–234, 1983.
8. Waitzkin H, Britt T. Processing narratives of self-destructive behavior in routine medical encounters: health promotion, disease prevention, and the discourse of health care. *Soc Sci Med* 36:1121–1136, 1993.
9. Ley P. Doctor-patient communication: Some quantitative estimates of the role of cognitive factors in non-compliance. *J Hypertens* 3:51–55, 1985.
10. Waitzkin H. Doctor-patient communication: Clinical implications of social scientific research. *JAMA* 252:2441–2446, 1984.
11. Ley P. Memory for medical information. *Br J Soc Clin Psychol* 18:245–255, 1979.
12. Ley P, et al. Improving doctor-patient communication in general practice. *J R Coll Gen Pract* 26:720–724, 1976.

13. Quill TE, Townsend P. Bad news: delivery, dialogue, and dilemmas. *Arch Intern Med* 151:463–468, 1991.
14. Fallowfield LJ, Lipkin M. Delivering Sad or Bad News. In Lipkin M, Putnam SM, Lazare A (eds.), *The Medical Interview*. New York: Springer-Verlag, 1995. Pp. 316–323.
15. Williams GC, et al. "The facts concerning the recent carnival of smoking in Connecticut" and elsewhere. *Ann Intern Med* 115:59–63, 1991.

Appendix A

Examples of Some Emotions*

Abandoned
Afraid
Aggravated
Agitated
Alienated
Alive
Alone
Amazed
Ambiguous
Ambivalent
Amused
Angry
Annoyed
Anxious
Appalled
Apprehensive
Ashamed
Astounded
Astonished
At ease
Awed
Awkward

Bad
Bashful
Betrayed
Bitchy
Bitter
Blamed
Blissful
Blocked

Blue
Bored
Bothered
Bugged
Bummed-out
Burdened

Calm
Capable
Captivated
Cautious
Challenged
Charmed
Cheated
Cheerful
Childish
Clever
Combative
Comfortable
Committed
Compassionate
Concerned
Condemned
Confident
Conflicted
Confused
Consumed
Contented
Contrite
Controlled
Creative

Crummy
Crushed
Curious

Deceitful
Deceived
Defeated
Defiant
Degraded
Dejected
Delighted
Depressed
Despair
Destructive
Determined
Devastated
Different
Dirty
Disappointed
Discouraged
Disgusted
Disoriented
Dissatisfied
Distracted
Distraught
Distressed
Distrustful
Disturbed
Dominated
Doubtful
Down

Downtrodden
Drained
Driven
Dumb

Eager
Ecstatic
Edgy
Elated
Embarrassed
Empty
Encouraged
Energetic
Engrossed
Engulfed
Enlightened
Enraged
Enthusiastic
Envious
Euphoric
Evil
Exasperated
Excited
Exhausted

Fearful
Flustered
Foolish
Forgotten
Forlorn
Fragmented

217

Frantic	Independent	Modest	Rage
Frenzied	Indifferent	Morose	Refreshed
Fretful	Inferior	Mystified	Regretful
Friendly	Infuriated		Rejected
Frightened	Insecure	Needed	Rejuvenated
Frustrated	Insensitive	Negative	Relaxed
Funny	Inspired	Neglected	Relieved
Furious	Interested	Nervous	Remorseful
	Intimidated	Numb	Renewed
Gloomy	Involved	Nutty	Resentful
Glum	Irritated		Resigned
Good	Isolated	Obnoxious	Restless
Grateful		Obsessed	Rewarded
Gratified	Jealous	Odd	Righteous
Great	Jittery	Oppressed	Rotten
Grief	Joyful	Outraged	
Groovy	Jubilant	Overwhelmed	Sad
Grouchy	Jumpy		Safe
Guilty		Pained	Satisfied
Gullible	Lazy	Panicked	Scared
	Left out	Patient	Scattered
Happy	Let down	Peaceful	Screwed up
Hassled	Lethargic	Perplexed	Secure
Hateful	Lighthearted	Persecuted	Selfish
Helpful	Listless	Perturbed	Sensitive
Helpless	Lonely	Petrified	Sensuous
Hesitant	Longing	Phony	Serious
High	Loved	Picked on	Shattered
Hopeful	Loving	Pity	Shocked
Hopeless	Low	Pleasant	Shy
Horrible		Pleased	Smothered
Horrified	Mad	Positive	Solemn
Hostile	Manipulated	Pressured	Sophisticated
Hurt	Marvelous	Preoccupied	Sorrowful
	Maudlin	Proud	Sorry
Ignorant	Mean	Pushed	Spiteful
Ignored	Meek	Put down	Strange
Impatient	Melancholy	Put upon	Strong
Impulsive	Mellow	Puzzled	Stubborn
Important	Miserable		Stuck
Inadequate	Misunderstood	Quarrelsome	Stunned
Incompetent	Mixed up	Quiet	Stupefied

Stupid	Thwarted	Uncomfortable	Vital
Successful	Tired	Uneasy	Vivacious
Suffering	Tormented	Unfortunate	Vulnerable
Superfluous	Torn	Unhappy	
Superior	Tranquil	Unimportant	
Surprised	Trapped	Uninvolved	Warm
Suspicious	Tremendous	Unlucky	Weak
Sympathetic	Troubled	Unpleasant	Wary
	Tuned on	Unsettled	Weepy
	Turned off	Unwanted	Whimsical
Tense	Terrific	Upset	Whole
Tentative	Terrified	Uptight	Wicked
Terrible		Useful	Wonderful
Terrified		Useless	Worried
Testy	Ugly		Worthless
Threatened	Uncertain	Violent	Worthwhile

*Adapted from Coulehan JL, Block MR. *The Medical Interview: A Primer for Students of the Art.* Philadelphia: FA Davis, 1987.

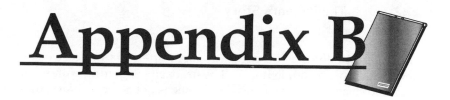

Appendix B

Write-Up of Mrs. Jones' Evaluation

Joanne Elizabeth Jones
Clinical Center #12 34 56
February 29, 1994

Identifying Data: This is the first visit to the Clinical Center for this 38-year-old married white woman who is a local attorney with GHI Corporation. The interview was obtained by J. White, a third-year medical student.

Source and Reliability of Information: The patient was cooperative and reliable. No other informants or data sources were available.

Chief Complaint/Agenda: The chief complaint is (1) Headaches in the context of problem (2): difficulties with her boss. Other agenda items are (3) cough, (4) "colitis," and (5) she wants to know if medications for colitis need to be added.

History of the Present Illness: The patient's headache began rather suddenly at work 3 months ago. Headaches were accompanied by nausea during the last month and she vomited once last week during the most severe headache ever, which prompted this appointment.

The headaches are located diffusely over the right temporal region and do not radiate elsewhere. They feel deep within the head, are not associated with tenderness or increased sensitivity of the scalp, and are described as pounding and throbbing. They begin suddenly and then increase in intensity, described as "worse than having a baby" when severe. Mrs. Jones has had to miss work a few days because of the intense pain. The headaches occur two to three times per week and can last as long as 12 hours at a time,

221

although initially they occurred no more often than once weekly and lasted only a couple hours. The headache is getting worse but seems to clear on the weekends when she is not at work. Nevertheless, the headaches have progressively worsened and are interfering with her life. Bright lights make the headache worse (photophobia). Lying in a dark room and placing an ice bag on her head seem to help. Drinking wine also may have been a precipitant once or twice. Nausea accompanies all headaches and she vomited a small amount of nonbloody material with one severe headache a week ago. The patient feels entirely well between her spells of headache and nausea.

Except for a problem of being carsick a couple times as a youngster, there have been no other associated symptoms in neurological, gastrointestinal, or other body systems. In particular, there has been no loss of consciousness, change in vision, paralysis, stiff neck, rash, fever, chills, change in memory, or history of seizures. She feels well otherwise, has a good appetite, and enjoys outside activities. There is no history of joint pain or swelling.

An injection in the emergency room 1 week ago provided relief, but the exact medication is not yet known to us; only a blood and urine test were obtained, the results of which are not yet available. Except for no more than six to eight aspirin daily and this one injection, she takes nothing for the headaches and has seen no other caretakers. Regarding possible causative factors, she has been taking birth control pills for 6 years and there is a possible history of migraine in an aunt. There is no history of head injury or neck injury.

Mrs. Jones' headaches occur at times of conflict with her boss. She is the corporation's new lead attorney and was brought in to replace the man who is now her boss, and promised there would be no problem during a year of transition prior to his retirement. He has been pushing and criticizing her, which makes her angry, and this leads to the headaches. She is also angry at the Board for promising that this problem would not occur. The relationship of anger and headache is similar to what she experienced as a child when her mother would unfairly criticize her. She believes her boss is the problem because, when she can avoid him, she has no headaches. She wants help with the headaches and coping with the stress because she is afraid they will adversely affect her and her family's personal lives. She is considering leaving her job. She has friends who provide support at work and her husband is supportive, but he doesn't say much because he encouraged her to take the job.

Health Issues

Ethical-Social-Spiritual Issues

1. Mrs. Jones has never considered advance directives. She and her husband have arranged for power of attorney, but she does not think it includes directions for health issues.
2. She wants to resume church activities, which have faltered during the last few years as life got busier, but, she says, "I don't want all that guilt stuff." Mrs. Jones indicates that her children have brought her more meaning in life than anything else, and that she and her husband are often able to "get out of ourselves" through them.

Functional Status

Mrs. Jones has no functional limitations.

Health-Promoting and Health-Maintenance Activities

1. The patient adheres carefully to a low-fat, low-salt diet and exercises actively in an aerobics class four to five times weekly for 45 minutes or so; this is vigorous enough to bring the pulse rate to 150 beats per minute and prompt a drenching sweat. Her weight is stable in the 120-pound range. She always uses her seat belt but does not have air-bags or antilock brakes. She does not ride bicycles or motorcycles, there are no weapons in the home, all medications are out of reach of the children, and the furnace is checked yearly for carbon monoxide emissions. She would like to take time for relaxation but does not do so now. She enjoys painting but worries that she is getting so busy that it will fall into the background. She describes herself as a "workaholic" and says that this prevents her from doing more interesting things like her painting, but that it does not keep her away from her children. She would like to curtail her work activities but sees no way to do this now in a busy new job. She and her husband also "socialize" a lot. Although neither seems to enjoy it much, it is part of their businesses and she sees no alternatives.
2. She has had regular physical examinations, including a Pap smear one year ago, with Dr. Jergens, who has also been her primary care physician; she does not know what blood tests he performed but some were done. She thinks her cholesterol was normal when hospitalized in 1982. She has not seen a dentist since a cavity was filled 4 years ago, although she has no

symptoms. She examines her breasts regularly about a week after each menstrual period.

3. She has had all of the usual "baby shots" but does not know exactly what they were. A tetanus shot was given 2 years ago following a puncture wound to the hand. She does not think flu shots work and does not want anymore because she got sick after the last one 3 years ago.

Health Hazards

1. Except for a rare cup of coffee and glass of wine, the patient has not used addicting substances.
2. The patient and her husband are monogamous and heterosexual. She had two other sexual partners prior to marriage. There is no history of sexually transmitted diseases or of sexual abuse. Mrs. Jones has been satisfied with her sexual life until the last 3 months when her interest has decreased and her husband has had problems with inconstant impotence. Sexual intercourse now occurs about once weekly, but was three to four times weekly before starting this job. She is not worried about this, thinks that it relates to her work problems, and was not interested in further discussing it.
3. There is no history of physical or sexual abuse directed toward Mrs. Jones nor has she ever been abusive.

Past Medical History

Hospitalizations

1. 1982—She was hospitalized for 3 days and a diagnosis of mild ulcerative colitis was made. She presented with a 3-month history of periodic loose stools with occasional blood and mild abdominal cramping. Tests for "parasites and other germs" were negative at the University Hospital in the city where she was attending law school. She was cared for by a Dr. Jergens. Sigmoidoscopy and barium enema led to the diagnosis of ulcerative colitis and she was told she didn't need surgery but to follow-up closely, which she did at about 6-month intervals. She took prednisone for the first 3 months following discharge, starting at 40 mg daily and slowly reducing the dosage. She also took sulfasalazine, starting at 8 tablets daily (presumably 500-mg tablets but not yet verified). After 3 months, when the prednisone was stopped, the dose of sulfasalazine was slowly reduced to 4 tablets daily over the ensuing 3 months. This was stopped altogether a year later. She was

asymptomatic until November 1991 when some diarrhea without blood developed. Sigmoidoscopy by Dr. Jergens showed a mild flare-up and a barium enema showed only minor changes in the "distal sigmoid colon." Again, no surgery was advised and she was treated with sulfasalazine (she brought this pharmacy label), 1.0 g qid. for about 2 months. It was then gradually reduced to 0.5 g qid. for 6 months and then stopped. There has been no recurrence of symptoms. At her most recent sigmoidoscopy with Dr. Jergens 6 months ago, she was told her colon looked essentially normal and that nothing further was necessary except close follow-up.
2. Two uncomplicated obstetric confinements 6 and 8 years ago, produced healthy children. She was hospitalized less than 72 hours each time.
3. Tonsillectomy and adenoidectomy as a child.

Other Medical, Surgical, or Psychological Problems
1. As noted, she followed up regularly with Dr. Jergens for her ulcerative colitis and he also acted as her primary physician until she moved here 5 months ago, since which time she has seen no one except for one emergency room visit. Dr. Jergens urged her to get a primary care physician when she moved here.
2. Cough and stuffy nose 3 weeks ago with a slight persisting cough. There was no sore throat, ear ache, or fever and the cough is nearly gone. She took an over-the-counter cough medication for a week at the beginning, but doesn't recall the name.
3. Her first and only episode of urinary tract infection occurred in July 1993 with symptoms of increased frequency and dysuria. She felt well otherwise and there was no hematuria, fever, chills, or back pain. She received a 7-day course of trimethoprim/sulfamethoxazole tablets (twice daily) from an emergency room in Colorado, where they were vacationing, and was symptom-free within 2 days.
4. Fracture of left ulna 21 years ago as the result of a fall. It was casted for several weeks and there has been no problem since.
5. Knows she had measles and chicken pox as child and thinks she had a mild case of the mumps.

Screen for Major Diseases
1. There is no history of rheumatic fever, scarlet fever, diabetes mellitus, cancer, tuberculosis, heart disease, venereal disease, or stroke.

2. She has never received blood transfusions, insulin, digitalis, blood thinners, heart medications, or blood pressure medications.

Medications and Other Treatments

1. Aspirin, 6 to 8 five-grain tablets daily with her headaches during the last 4 to 6 weeks, with smaller amounts during the preceding 6 weeks. No adverse effect.
2. "Birth control pill" of uncertain type. She will call in the dosage and type.
3. No use of laxatives, vitamins, other hormones, nerve pills, tonics, or over-the-counter medications.
4. Except for Dr. Jergens, she has seen no one else and has not sought care from alternative healers. Nor does she use any nontraditional healing remedies.

Allergies and Drug Reactions

1. There is no history of allergies to drugs or other drug reactions.
2. There is no known allergic disease and no history of asthma, hives, or hay fever.
3. There is no known food or environmental substance to which she is sensitive.

Menstrual and Obstetric History

1. Menses began at age 12 and are attended by only slight discomfort for a day or so. They last 5 days, require 5 pads daily, and occur regularly every month since she has been on the birth control pill.
2. She is gravida (pregnancies) 2, para (deliveries) 2, abortus (spontaneous and induced abortions) 0, with 2 healthy living children. There have been no complications of her pregnancies, both vaginal deliveries.

Social History

Current Personal Situation

The patient is 38 years old and just moved here with her husband and two children 5 months ago. She left a job as a corporate attorney in the city where she had trained as a lawyer to come here with GHI Corporation as the lead attorney. See the HPI.

She views her new job here as a big professional step upward in corporate law. It provides the opportunity for leadership and creativity that didn't exist previously. Her husband also is a lawyer with GHI but works in a different area. His job was a big step upward for him as well; he is quite happy here and is getting along well. Both were happy in their previous jobs but felt the need to progress professionally.

She has no financial problems and is well covered by health insurance.

Other Personal Factors

The patient was born in a small farming community in Kansas on 8-12-55. There was one younger sibling, a brother born 3-14-58. Her parents were her primary caretakers although her father's parents lived in the area and frequently assisted in raising the two children. Her father owned the local hardware store and the family had no financial problems but was not wealthy, described as "pretty much middle class." Her father was a loving, caring man but "always at work." She had a good relationship with him and frequently helped him out in the store. By the time she was in her teens, she could run the store in his absence. Her mother was "more critical" and always pushing her to do more things. She was insistent that the patient do well in school, not date boys with no future, and that she go to college. Her mother frequently lamented not having gone to college but was described as "very bright, but clever and biting in things she said." The patient never felt as close to her mother as to her father but nonetheless got along well with her, always understood what she wanted, and "knew that she loved me." She loved her younger brother greatly and they always had a special relationship, which continues to this day. She scarcely knew her mother's parents but grew up with her paternal grandparents close by, developing a very close relationship with her grandmother who was "very loving and accepting."

Her kindergarten through twelfth-grade schooling occurred in the same small town; there were about 100 students in her graduating high-school class. She did well in school, was well liked, and had many extracurricular activities. She dated frequently but never had a steady boyfriend or close relationship. The patient and her family attended church but "weren't very religious."

It was difficult to leave many friends and family when she went off to college far from home on scholarship. She recalls "moping around" for several weeks but then getting over it as she got into the flow of school and began to meet other new students. She did well in school and graduated 4 years later. During college, she had two serious relationships, including sexual activity, but in both cases decided against marriage because of her desire to go to law school and forgo a family.

She attended law school at the same university and did extremely well. She also periodically resumed one of the close relationships above during this time but didn't want to marry as her boyfriend did. She preferred to date casually and attend to her studies.

She began working with a large, prestigious law firm in the same city following graduation in 1980. She slowly worked her way up to a midlevel position in their hierarchy and was happy until the last year or so when she realized she would never have the chance for the independence and creativity that she wanted.

She met her husband at work in 1981 and they were married in 1982 after her colitis cleared. He had similar professional values and ideas about children, and she describes their relationship as very compatible, until the current problems with their sexual lives. Their oldest son was born in 1985 and the second son was born in 1987. She describes her children as "the best thing I ever did" and said they give her life real meaning. She was "quite happy and satisfied" with life "until I got here." She has several friends at work and locally.

Family History

General and Specific Inquiry

There are no known diseases the patient is aware of that seem to run in the family and, in particular, the patient is aware of no familial problems with the following: tuberculosis, cancer, heart disease, bleeding problems, kidney failure, dialysis, alcoholism, tobacco use, weight problems, asthma, or mental illness. Her paternal grandmother has diabetes mellitus.

Genogram

Figure B-1 is an example of Mrs. Jones' genogram.

Review of Systems (System Review)

General: nothing additional
Integument: had rash while traveling that seemed due to harsh soaps; no recurrence since moving here
Hematopoietic: excessive bruising years ago when taking prednisone but none since

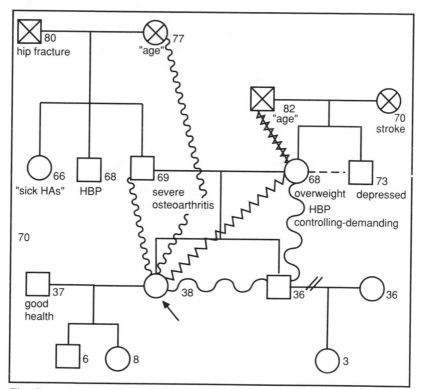

Fig. B-1. Mrs. Jones' genogram. Age of family members appears to the right of each. Under some figures is listed the cause of death (deceased persons) or the current status of living persons. Key: □ = male; ○ = female; ⊠ = deceased; —//—= divorced; ⌒⌒⌒ = close (good) relationship; ⋀⋀⋀⋀ = conflicted relationship; ⋀⋀⋀⋀= close and conflicted relationship; ⋯⋯⋯ = distant relationship; ◄— = the patient; HBP = high blood pressure; HA = headaches. (Mullins HC, Christie-Seely J. Collection and recording family data: the geogram. In Christie-Seely J (ed.), *Working with the Family in Primary Care: A Systems Approach to Health and Illness.* New York: Praeger, 1984. Pp. 179–191. Reprinted with permission of Greenwood Publishing Group, Inc., Westport, CT. Copyright © 1984.)

Endocrine: nothing additional
Musculoskeletal: nothing additional
Eyes, Ears, Nose, Throat: uses reading glasses when doing much reading
Head and Neck: nothing additional
Breasts: breasts are generally "lumpy" around her periods but never has felt any masses. Did not nurse her children

Cardiovascular and Pulmonary: nothing additional
Gastrointestinal: nothing additional except moderately painful hemorrhoids in the later stages of each pregnancy
Urinary: nothing additional except for brief period of enuresis around age 5
Genital: nothing additional
Neuropsychiatric: nothing additional

Physical Examination*
Because this text does not address the physical examination, we will only summarize pertinent findings. Suffice it to say that Mrs. Jones had a blood pressure of 110/70, a pulse rate of 66, and 12 respirations per minute. There was no evidence of neurological or gastrointestinal abnormality; these are the areas most likely to have explanatory value for her symptoms if abnormalities were found. Except for a midsystolic click along the left sternal border heard on auscultation of the heart (suggests mitral valve prolapse), there were no other abnormalities on physical examination either.

Initial Diagnostic and Treatment Interventions*
None

Assessment: Biopsychosocial Description —
The Patient's Story**

Relationship Story
STUDENT'S RESPONSES
1. Liked her and felt good about her compliments.
2. Uncomfortable when she spoke of her sexual problems and might have cut the conversation short.
3. Uneasy not knowing more about diseases that cause headaches.

MRS. JONES' PERSONALITY STYLE
Minor obsessive features within the range of normal.

INTERACTION
1. Warm and respectful. The patient made good eye contact and indicated several times that she valued the work.

*Included for completeness but not addressed in this book.
**Included for completeness but not addressed in this book except to note how assessments are made using the RPD method of recording. Many supervisors request that the Assessment or Problem List contain extensive discussion of the student's reasoning as well as a comprehensive review of the literature about the problem.

2. The patient developed a headache while discussing problems involving her boss and her mother.

[Note how subsequent personal and disease dimensions interact with the relational.]

Personal Story

1. Severe stress from a critical boss, resulting in anger (closely associated with headaches) at him and the Board that recruited her.
2. Similar relationship of headaches and anger since childhood, in response to a critical mother.

[Note how her personal story interacts with her disease and relational story.]

Disease Story

BIOMEDICAL

1. Intermittent right temporal headaches, throbbing, associated with nausea and photophobia, increasing in frequency and severity over 3 months, on birth control pills, associated with severe stress, and without historical or physical exam evidence of neurological dysfunction. The following are the diagnostic possibilities, in order of likelihood:
   a. migraine headache,
   b. stress-tension headache,
   c. chronic meningitis—very unlikely,
   d. vasculitis; e.g., systemic lupus erythematosus—very unlikely, or
   e. chronic subdural hematoma—very unlikely.
2. Nausea with one episode of vomiting—Most likely part of the above picture.
3. Recent respiratory tract infection ("cold"), cleared.
4. Idiopathic ulcerative colitis, quiescent and mild by her report.
5. Past history of one lower urinary tract infection 8 months ago.
6. Probable mitral valve prolapse, asymptomatic and likely of no clinical importance.

PSYCHIATRIC

None

[Note the interaction of the disease aspects with the personal dimension and relational dimension.]

Treatment and Investigative Plan*

Headaches
1. Obtain records from recent emergency room visit.
2. Start treatment of migraine headaches with ergotamine tartrate and caffeine tablets.
3. Will consider later addition of prophylactic treatment with a beta blocker or calcium channel blocker if 2 is not effective.
4. Also, will need to consider discontinuing the birth control pill and finding an alternative means of contraception if 2 and 3 are not effective.
5. Defer any investigation of the headaches until observing the impact of treatment on what appears to be typical migraine.
6. Further discuss specific strategies for dealing with her boss at the next visit in 1 week.
7. Instruct her in a relaxation procedure.

Ulcerative Colitis
1. Obtain outside records for Dr. Jergens.
2. Flexible sigmoidoscopy.

Index

Note: Page numbers followed by *f* indicate figures; those followed by *t* indicate tables.